The Life of Riley

Mastering the five secret habits to enjoy a longer and healthier life

Phil Riley MBA

Published by Columbus Publishing Ltd 2016
www.columbuspublishing.co.uk

ISBN 978-1-907797-50-7
Version 20160422

Cover design by Lewis Kokoc

Author portrait by Emilie Sandy

Brand and product names are trademarks or registered trademarks of their respective owners.

The content of this book is intended to inform, entertain and provoke your thinking. This is not intended as medical advice. It may, however, make you question current medical and nutritional advice. That's your choice. It's your life and health in your hands.
Neither the author nor the publisher can be held responsible or liable for any loss or claim arising from the use, or misuse, of the content of this book.

COLUMBUS PUBLISHING

Acknowledgements

I would first like to thank Zoë and Andy Harcombe, for having the faith to publish *The Life of Riley*. As another publisher said to me, I am neither a celebrity, nor a scientist, so I'm starting at the back of the field as far as health books go. Therefore my particular story, and my take on the science and practicalities of extending your healthy life expectancy, needed a champion, and Zoë & Andy fitted that bill.

As you'll discover, the genesis of the book is radio, and I'd like to thank everyone who has helped me enjoy such a great career in this wonderful business, and the many terrific friends and colleagues I have made during my time in broadcasting.

On the statistics, and my modelling, I am grateful to the doyenne of UK radio research, Rachel Steel, for checking I haven't made any arithmetical or statistical blunders. The analysis and conclusions though are mine, not hers, to criticise. Thanks too go to former radio colleagues Daniel Owen and Paul Fairburn for also helping proof-read and check. Geoff Percy was an early convert too, and his advice and support has been invaluable, as has the support of long-time friends John Myers and Simon Cole.

A special thank you also to Jonathan Dean for all his hard work and expertise in helping set up thelifeofrileybook.com website.

My three children, Alex, Jess and Matt all share some of the blame for *The Life of Riley*. They have long nagged me over my drinking, but it wasn't until they'd left home that I got the peace and quiet to really figure out the various strands of the book – as well as curtail my wine consumption.

Finally my biggest thanks go to my wife Jean. She has not only suffered through my smoking, bad eating habits, lack of fitness and over-indulgence in alcohol, but she has stuck with me as I've attempted to fix those shortcomings, one by one. She also came with me on the plan itself, once it was created in the summer of 2014, and probably sticks to it more religiously than I, if I'm honest. Truly you are my better half.

Contents

Note

The phrase "The Life of Riley" originated as a lyric in a song in the 1880s, and has gradually come into common usage to describe someone living a carefree, idyllic lifestyle, free from concerns or worries.

If you follow the habits outlined in this book, I can't promise you a completely carefree life, but I think you should end up with far fewer worries and more happiness – certainly about your life expectancy and health.

I've always been secretly pleased my surname has been tied to this particular phrase, and it's great to be able to use it as this book's title.

I was also delighted when The Lightning Seeds used it as the title to one of their best-known songs (the instrumental break in the track has been used extensively in *Match of The Day*) and I used it as the play-out song for my mum's funeral. She would have been amused.

Foreword

Average life expectancy has been increasing pretty steadily over the last 30 years, by around 2 years every decade. There's no reason to think this increase will slow down anytime soon.

In fact, receiving a telegram on your 100th birthday used to be so rare as to make a story in the local paper. Not these days. More and more of us are living to 100 or even longer. 1% of men, and almost 3% of women can now expect that message from the Queen. Amazingly, in 2014, over 7,500 telegrams were sent to men and women who had lived through two world wars.

Yet many of us are also dying far younger than we need to.

No one can guarantee the age they will live to, but there is mounting scientific evidence that a few, simple lifestyle changes can add years to your life and dramatically increase your chances of living to a ripe old-age.

And those lifestyle changes also make you more likely to be able to enjoy your later years in better physical and mental health.

I'm not going to spend any time in this book discussing the rather horrible ways people can, and do, die if they live poor lifestyles. You probably already know most of them, and being reminded of them is not necessarily helpful in trying to get your mind round actually doing something about it. So, apart from a very brief summary of the problems associated with the four deadly lifestyle habits I will outline later, I'll leave the blood and gore to government health campaigns – they seem to specialise in that sort of thing.

I will, however, take you through those lifestyle challenges in this book, and explain why adopting five new habits could mean decades being added to your healthy life expectancy.

I'll also explain why your later life doesn't need to be lived in the shadow of ill-health and inconvenience.

Amazingly, in looking at all the mounds of information available on lifestyle choices and their effects on health and mortality, the bad effects of poor choices are well documented, but the reverse – the good effects of avoiding poor choices – is nowhere to be found. Until now.

If this were a business problem to be solved, with the chance to make money at the end, companies would be falling over themselves to offer solutions to help people move away from poor lifestyle choices and towards a lifestyle that could maximise their longevity. And treating this as a business problem to be solved using the basics of good management is how I've approached this book.

And I think you will be amazed when I show you what the statistics actually say can be achieved by ordinary people like you and me who even modestly manage to change how we live.

A few words on science and business

In my day job of broadcasting, our journalism has to abide by strict rules on honesty, fairness, accuracy and impartiality. In business too, you simply can't pull the wool over people's eyes and try to con them into buying your product. You will get found out quickly enough if you aren't offering good value for money. You have to be honest, upfront and offer a real benefit if you want to succeed (although, given the antics of some car companies recently, maybe I'm being a little naïve on this point).

I have tried to apply these rules of honesty, fairness and value to my reporting and analysis of the data, statistics and science that underpin much of this book. Because of this I have followed a few simple rules.

As I am writing about western lifestyles, and how they impact on longevity, I have tended to only use western research wherever possible – particularly research and data from the USA, UK, Western Europe and the wider Anglosphere. Developing countries have a different set of lifestyle issues, which are outside the scope of this book.

A recent widely-reported study about the ease with which unscrupulous people can distort and alter research to generate misleading media coverage (*"Eating chocolate can help as part of weight loss[i]"*) shows how easy it can be to manipulate science to create a partial narrative for commercial or reputational gain. That is certainly not my intention here.

Because of this, I have tended to use meta-data and meta-analysis wherever it has been available. For those unfamiliar, this is the technique whereby scientists bring together multiple studies, and add up larger amounts of data to see if these bigger samples can show clearer trends or patterns. This approach eliminates much of the bias that can (either intentionally or unintentionally) occur in smaller, one-off pieces of research.

Where meta-analysis hasn't been available I have tried to use the best, most current research publicly available. I have tended to use studies either from governments or from the more prestigious institutions if possible, so Harvard, or Cambridge, for example, feature more heavily than other, lesser-known bodies. I know this isn't perfect, and the largest and most prestigious bodies can also occasionally get things wrong (as of course can governments), but you have to start somewhere.

If I have been able to find multiple studies to support an assertion I will have referenced them.

Much of what I propose in this book is actually fairly undisputed. I think most scientists would find little to argue with in many of my conclusions. However, there are still raging disagreements in a number of areas. To give just three examples:

What are the benefits of vaping?

Which of low-carb or low-fat diets is more effective?

Is there an "ideal" weight?

Where there is a debate, I have quoted what I think is the best available research and then moved on to make my own conclusions based on reading both sides of the argument.

And some questions have so much conflicting science right now I think they are currently impossible to answer definitively (what is a safe level of alcohol to consume, for example). Here I have just taken the latest research and caveated accordingly.

In some instances, I have wanted to use some research which has been reported on, but where the original data has not been easy to source and refer to. In these cases I have used the reporting as my reference, but only where the story has appeared in a newspaper of record such as *The New York*

Times, Times of London, The Guardian etc.

I am not a scientist reporting back on my experimental findings here (or a celebrity selling a pre-Christmas blockbuster on my transformational lifestyle change to raise my profile) so my approach to this issue has been to tackle the problem of increasing longevity, healthily, from a business perspective, i.e. what is the problem and how can we solve it in the most efficient way.

Business is an art, not a science. It is practical, not theoretical. However, good business planning is now more structured than ever before, and there are well-trodden paths to success. Clear and accurate problem identification; good research into root causes; analysis of target demographics; quantitative modelling; plan creation and testing; benefits marketing – all great industry jargon – but representative of real thinking and good problem solving.

I've tried to apply some of the basics of business thinking and practical problem solving to this journey into life expectancy. Where a particular business concept has been used, I've simply tagged it in the main section of the book and expanded upon it in Appendix 2. If you are a business fan you can read the appendix to gain greater understanding – but if management jargon puts you off you can simply skip that end-section altogether. Whatever your views on business, I hope you enjoy *The Life of Riley* habits which emerged.

Chapter 1

"This strange and mournful day"

Mother & Child Reunion – Paul Simon

2013 came as quite a shock to me.

Three friends and former work colleagues died in relatively quick succession during the year[1]. Now people die all the time, but the shock here was that two were in their fifties, and one in his mid-sixties.

I've worked for 35 years in the radio business, and although we have a lot of fun, I wouldn't say we were any more dissolute as a group of people than other professions. But three guys I knew, who I would have considered contemporaries in terms of age (I was 54 at the time) dying within six months of each other came as a real wake up call, both to me and I'm sure those colleagues of mine who also had to keep digging their sombre clothes out of the wardrobe during that period.

We are constantly being told in the media that average life expectancy these days is 79[2], and whenever I ask people

---

[1] Dave Hickman was a presenter on both BRMB/Xtra AM and Heart – he died in July 2013, aged 54.
Bobby Williams was a Sales Exec and then manager at BRMB, Buzz FM and other local Birmingham stations. He died in October 2013 aged 59.
Mike Baker was a DJ/Presenter on Beacon Radio and Heart. He died in December 2013 aged 65.

[2] This is the correct number for total population (male + female) average (mean) life expectancy 0-100 (i.e. excluding those who live beyond 101) according to ONS data for life expectancy 2010-2012.
When all adults including those 101+ are added, the average (mean) rises to 80.9.

what they think life expectancy is, this is the figure most often quoted back at me, so my three mates losing 15 to 25 years off this average came as something of a shock. And by the way, 79 is actually not the best way of describing adult UK life expectancy. The real average adult life expectancy is significantly older, as I'll explain later.

Just before my friends and colleagues died, my mum had passed on, in May 2013, aged 77. Now my mum was a woman who had lived a challenging life, and had survived long enough to see me do alright for myself (she did keep asking me though, when I was an up and coming radio DJ in my 20s, when I was going to get a proper job), but although I loved her like any son loves their mum, I can't honestly say she had made the right lifestyle choices throughout her life. She was a heavy smoker, who had worked hard, but never exercised. She died of emphysema. In the end, she needed round the clock care, and although she was living in a lovely care home just two miles from our house, she spent a lot of her time outside, attempting to smoke herself to death, as the illness was so debilitating.

It was tragic to watch and be a part of.

Then I almost killed myself.

It happened on June 22nd 2013, the day of the first British and Irish Lions rugby test match in Australia, and I think the story is worth retelling.

That evening, my wife Jean and I were due to host a charity sporting dinner at my son Matt's school. 250 parents and friends were coming. I had organised the quiz, silent auction and guest speaker. Jean had sorted catering, the raffle, tables, money etc.. Lots of early prep came to a halt at 11am, as we settled down to watch the rugby.

Half time came, and Jean nipped out to pick up some last minute items for the dinner. She called from the car *"...lots of neighbours have the flags out – Union Jacks – we should put ours up..."*

Now I realise the Union Jack is not quite the right flag for the British and Irish Lions – but it's the thought that counts. So, game paused, I went out into the garden. The flagpole was there when we bought the house, and we do stick a St Georges Cross or Union Jack up for big sporting events. I grabbed the flag from the shed and proceeded to hoist it. At this point it got stuck and I needed to go back to the house to grab a stepladder to untangle it.

Back with the ladder... Just up a few feet... stretch up to grab the flag... a gust of wind... slightly knocking me off balance... the stepladder shifts slightly as one of the legs sinks into a spot of soft ground... I lose my balance ever so slightly... I grab the flagpole to keep myself upright as I fall off the ladder... I sink to the floor still holding on to the pole, only a few feet down... I realise I have a sharp pain in my forearm... and I look up to see my forearm skewered on the cleat, the metal prong which you loop the rope around... I am well and truly skewered too, and have to physically lift my arm off the cleat as I get back up on my feet.

I then look at my forearm. It is completely ripped open, exposing tendons, muscle, bone etc. It's a truism in life that if you can see your insides, you are not in a good place. I was not in a good place.

That scene in *The Terminator*, where Arnie slices open his forearm – it was just like that, except there were no steel rods or cables visible – just tendons and bones – I was mortifyingly human – and really exposed.

Not much blood though, I thought, as I gingerly grabbed my left arm in my right hand and walked quickly back to the house, hoping I wouldn't faint, or trip, as I went inside.

I shouted for Matt, and in I'm sure slightly overexcited tones asked him to call 999 and his mum *"...I'm not in a good place here son..."* I said, as I sat down, put a towel round my exposed flesh and thought of the many horrible outcomes that could befall me.

Jean got back in around 10 minutes. She looked as shocked as I felt. I've fallen off my bike a few times, incurring cuts and bruises, but this was something potentially far more serious, and we both knew it.

Keith and Kirsty were the paramedics who arrived shortly after. Keith an experienced, calm health professional. Kirsty younger, learning the ropes. Keith calmed me down and tested my fingers and wrist for damage.

Amazingly, there didn't seem to be anything wrong mechanically. In what must rank as one of the luckiest escapes ever, I appeared to have missed slicing anything important. I could squeeze, push etc. – although actually being able to see the tendons moving was hugely unnerving. At this point I just looked away. "Right..." said Keith "...if you want, we can sew you up here..."

"Go for it" I said. And so Keith and Kirsty proceeded to put 16 stitches into my arm on my dining room table, in full view of my wife and son, at 12.30pm on an otherwise unremarkable Saturday afternoon.

Out came the "Gas & Air" so frequently given to expectant mums starting childbirth. You women have kept this secret from us blokes for too long! Within seconds I was high as a kite. We were laughing and joking with each other as the sutures went in – nothing had ever seemed as funny as falling off that ladder, slicing my arm open, leaving the flag half erected. I laughed so much we needed a second tank of the gas! Or was it because putting 16 stitches into a six inch long wound just took so long?

1.30, and Keith and Kirsty were gone. They had lived up to every ideal we like to imagine health professionals strive for – cool, calm, courteous, professional, and good. Life savers.

2pm – dosed up with codeine, I am contemplating what this means.

In the short term, it means I can get the charity dinner sorted, which Jean and I do, me through gritted teeth and more painkillers. Never has a fun evening seemed so long and arduous! We raised £12,000 though, to help rebuild a school in Christchurch in NZ devastated by their recent earthquake. Job done, we left just after midnight – as bone tired as we've ever been.

During the first two days after the accident, everyone I met told me I looked pale and shocked. And that's because I was. Given how tightly I was gripping the flagpole, completely unaware of the damage I was about to do, I was maybe half an inch away from tearing into muscle and/or tendon, severely damaging my left, dominant arm, causing me a lifetime of pain and inconvenience. More worryingly, I was also half an inch from tearing open my Radial or Ulnar artery. And that's what haunts me. I could easily have bled out, lying by a stupid flag pole, on an otherwise perfectly normal, boring Saturday, with no-one knowing quite where I was, my wife out doing errands, my son a few hundred yards away, watching rugby on the TV.

It isn't very often you come that close to your own mortality and live to tell the tale – but I did.

So, in 2013 I saw three friends die in their 50s and early 60s, I watched my mum pass away in a horrible death, and I ended up with a bloody big scar in a near-fatal accident, aged 54. What did it all mean?

As the clock ticked round at the end of the year I had started to wonder far more deeply about the nature of life, and how it can be taken away from us so easily. I resolved to take more care of myself, and I also decided to ask myself a few questions, in exactly the way I would if faced with a problem at work.

- What was it about lifestyle that was causing so many premature deaths, and how easy was it to change?

- Could you change at any stage? I was 54 and considered myself in good shape, but if I was still doing something wrong, I wanted to know about it, and whether it was worth changing?

- What was the real number for life expectancy? As I'd just seen 4 people die in their 50s, 60s and 70s, and the average was supposedly 79, did that mean there were an equivalent number of folk still around into their 80s, 90s and beyond?

- Was living that long just good luck (or all in your genes), or was there something positive you could do with your lifestyle to increase your chances of getting to this age?

- If lifestyle was the answer, then even if I could figure out a way to change bad lifestyle habits, could I do it successfully, and stick with it over a long period?

I decided then and there to try and answer those questions by applying the same practical, questioning and structured approach to problem solving which had served me so well throughput my business career. Was there an efficient "business solution" to longevity issues – and if so could I capture it and write it down, thereby creating my own personal "business plan" for extending life expectancy? And if I could do that, why not share it?

Hence this book.

Chapter 2

"The lights are turning red"

Life in the fast lane – Eagles

One of my favourite management gurus is Peter Drucker. His name will crop up frequently, along with some of his best quotes. He was a great believer in ensuring individuals who were embarking on a business career looked after themselves, so let's start with this comment from 1993.

"Only you can keep yourself healthy. That's new talk. It's old wisdom."

War, Famine, Pestilence and Death are the original Four Horsemen of the Apocalypse – characters named in *Revelations*, one of the books in The Bible, who are set to appear during the end-times. Story-telling is a particular theme in business – does an individual, or a brand, have a narrative tale that people can follow and identify with. I'm not big on religion myself, but the story-telling contained within it is very impactful, and the imagery surrounding these four characters is very powerful indeed, and of course their use as allegories is widespread, and I intend to continue that cliché in a moment.

If you are going to solve a problem in business, you first need to analyse what the problem actually is. And in my case, if you are going to try to figure out how to help people (including yourself) live longer, you first need to ask what people are dying of.

Most deaths in the advanced, western economies can be categorised into three different groups. In England &

Wales, where we are pretty good at recording these things, the data highlights the size of these three biggies; circulatory diseases (heart attacks, strokes, haemorrhages etc.) are top, and account for just under 33% of all deaths; cancers (prostate, breast, lung, stomach/digestive organs being the most prevalent) are next, at just under 30%; and respiratory diseases (influenza, pneumonia, emphysema etc.) are third, at around 14%[ii].

These three main causes trigger three quarters of all deaths in England & Wales. Every other cause is trivial in comparison. Although the absolute numbers will vary slightly I'm sure, I would expect the data to show very similar patterns across the western world.

[For the record, accidents account for 3.5% of all deaths. Not much we can do to predict these, and I'm going to pretty much ignore accidental death from now on in this book. But I'd urge you to be safe, and seriously, take care on ladders.]

Now an individual can of course die from one of these three big disease groups while living a perfectly blameless life. After all, a cancer is essentially a random act – a single cell mutating out of control, triggering other cells to do the same, and growing into a tumour. This can occur in anyone, at any time, through no fault of your own.

And anyone can catch pneumonia, or suffer a heart attack, no matter how physically active or healthy they appear to be, or have a genetic pre-disposition to cardio-vascular disease.

So all of the predictions and forecasts in this book are based on whole populations, not individuals. You may be more or less fortunate than others who live the same lifestyle as you, and at a personal level these things are impossible to predict.

However, as we all know, certain lifestyle decisions can increase the risk of our bodies succumbing to these random acts, and that is where the focus of this book lies: in identifying those lifestyle choices, and suggesting a simple, effective way of changing your life to avoid those, to be blunt, death-inducing selections.

My updated four horsemen, reaping mayhem on our bodies and health, are the four key lifestyle choices that we are making in the west in the 21st century that all the scientific evidence suggest are the leading causes of early mortality. Changing our approach to these is the key problem to be solved.

None of them will shock you.

They are:

- Heavy/frequent drinking
- Smoking
- Obesity
- Physical inactivity

Normally, in any business environment, once you have identified a problem which you think you could solve (for a profit of course) you would commission some research to identify the size of the market etc. Luckily for me, there already exists so much research into these lifestyles and their effect on life expectancy, my challenge was not to wait for any analysis I had commissioned myself to guide me to some answers, but to sift through the mounds of data already available to find the right solutions.

And this assertion, that these four lifestyle traits are the key to explaining vast differences in life expectancy, is backed up by overwhelming amounts of research, including most recently a comprehensive, ground-breaking study in Wales, Led by Professor Peter Elwood of Cardiff University, over a 35 year period, and following the lives of 2,500 men in South Wales (The Caerphilly Study)[iii].

The men who lived longest were the ones who

- Drank fewer than two glasses of wine a day;
- Didn't smoke;

- Stayed slim;
- Ate plenty of vegetables; and
- Exercised regularly.

Basically, the men who had avoided the scythes of my four horsemen lived longer. Anyone who had stuck with at least 4 of those lifestyle traits during the 35-year period was 60% less likely to have died since. They also suffered from 60% fewer heart attacks, 60% fewer cases of dementia, 40% fewer cancers and 70% fewer cases of diabetes.

Many of those who stuck to the habits were perfectly healthy well into their 80s and 90s.

This is just one, recent, local example of a slew of studies undertaken across the western world that show a clear connection between lifestyle and mortality.

However, the hidden downside of Professor Elwood's research is how few men stuck to these guidelines, even when they knew how effective they were. Only 5% managed to stick to four out of five of his habits, and only 1% to all five. I'll come back to this issue of "stickability" later in the book.

Now I am going to try to define these lifestyle choices quite carefully, because people can be forgiven for quitting early when faced with calls to embark on what they consider insuperable changes to how they live their lives, or think they are being told what to do by some "nanny state" bureaucrat. If I'm going to solve this problem, I can't begin by making the solution so unpalatable that collectively people simply reject the idea.

So, what I am <u>not</u> proposing in this book is that you need to become a stick-thin, super-fit triathlon participating, teetotal monk in order to live longer.

Far from it: in fact, based on the scientific evidence available, I think most people will be amazed at how little the shift needs to be in their lifestyle choices in order to dramatically increase their lifespan. Making the shift itself might not be easy, initially, but it genuinely won't be a huge shift for most people.

I want to be specific because in the next few chapters I then want to show you the effects of making these key decisions on your likely longevity.

One of the major issues we need to confront when discussing these lifestyle choices is both lack of awareness/information, and in many cases I'm afraid complete denial. In marketing terms this might best be described as making people aware of a "need" they didn't know they had.

This lack of knowledge or denial is evident across the piece:

- When asked, the level of drinking we say we are doing is significantly lower than the level of drinking recorded by alcohol sales, and many of us are blissfully unaware about recommended limits – or know those that have been in place for the last 20 years were simply intelligent guesses and therefore were safe to ignore.
- Social smokers consider themselves immune from the damage caused by cigarettes, despite strong evidence they are putting themselves at almost as high a risk as full-time smokers.
- A high proportion of people who are overweight or clinically obese consider themselves perfectly normal, and/or content with their weight.
- When asked, a majority of the population consider themselves to be fit, yet only one in five actually does enough physical activity to warrant that claim.

Let's look at those lifestyle choices in just a little more detail.

Heavy/Frequent Drinking:

We all think we know what alcoholism looks like. Down &

outs on the streets, begging for coins to feed their addiction, or family lives ruined by (usually) men who simply cannot control their craving for booze and veer off the normal path through life.

The recent tragic death of high-profile UK politician Charles Kennedy from an alcohol-related illness aged just 55 provoked a welcome public debate on attitudes to the illness, with well informed comment being led by Charles' friend and Tony Blair's former director of Communications Alistair Campbell, himself a self-confessed alcoholic, although someone who has now been dry for 18 years. And clearly this physical and mental addiction is an illness, and deserves to be treated as such, and is not the subject of this book. Latest UK government statistics estimate just over 100,000 adults in the UK are being treated for alcoholism.

But the problem of heavy/frequent drinking is a far larger one than the narrow focus on alcoholism. Even using the phrase "alcohol dependency" to capture a wider pool of at-risk folk is a potential problem in accurately describing this issue, as it implies some degree of addiction, which many people will feel is something they don't suffer from – even if at the same time they are drinking too much.

But whether you are severely addicted, mildly dependent, or simply an enthusiastic imbiber, your body will respond to the amount of alcohol consumed in exactly the same way.

So let's ignore whether you consider yourself dependent or not, and simply concentrate on the amount of alcohol you are consuming, and whether or not that level is safe.

Health professionals use a questionnaire known as the AUDIT test for those they think are at risk, and you can easily look this up online if you are curious[iv]. I will pose some questions for you in a moment on whether or not your drinking could be classed as "problematic" which are roughly based on a cut-down version of this test.

Heavy/frequent drinking means "sharing" a bottle of wine (or two) with your partner most nights of the week, or ensuring you regularly (i.e. virtually every night) stop off for a few pints to unwind after work. If this is you, then you are likely to be drinking at a level that will affect your long-term health.

Here are the three key questions.

1. How frequently do you drink each week? More than four nights a week regularly drinking is an indicator of risk.
2. How much are you consuming when you do drink? I'll discuss units later (arghh!) but for now, if you are a man and you are regularly drinking more than three pints or three medium glasses of wine per session, that is an indicator of risk. For a woman the figures will be regularly drinking more than two pints or two medium glasses.
3. Are any of these drinking occasions leading to excessive binge-drinking? If that is happening regularly, that is an indicator of risk too.

The acid test for me is that first question. Ask yourself, do you regularly go the majority of the week without drinking, or at least give yourself three nights drink-free? If you can't say yes to that question, you are at risk of cumulatively consuming more than is good for you and not giving your body any chance to recover, if you are combining it with significant amounts in each session.

For a man, 5 nights per week drinking 4 pints is 40 units – not quite alarm bells, but add in the extra drink or two at the weekend and you are getting mighty close. Similarly, a woman drinking 3 glasses of wine 5 nights a week is nudging 30 units. Weekend top-ups will again push her into concerning territory.

And that was my drinking behaviour up until a couple of years ago, so I think I know what a challenge this can be – so no judgements from me here.

The British Liver Trust recently did a study and showed that one in four of us was showing early signs of liver damage[v].

In fact, one amazing graph shows that, virtually alone amongst major diseases, only death from liver disease has risen in the UK over the past 40 years.

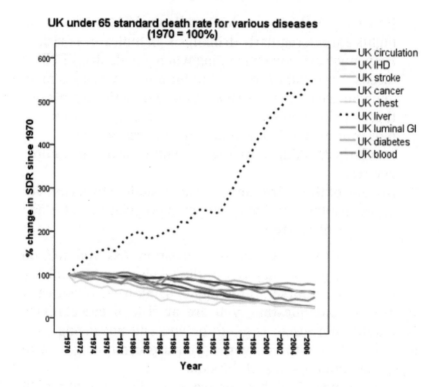

It's not just the booze at work here though. The sheer scale of this increase is in part due to non-alcoholic fatty liver disease[vi], which is separate to the damage being caused by alcohol. This disease is one of the new "hidden killers", affecting significant numbers of both obese and overweight people, and the combination of increased levels of drinking and increased obesity is the double whammy resulting in that massive spike in liver-related deaths.

In fact, although smoking is cumulatively the biggest factor in shortening life expectancy across the population as a whole, alcohol dependency is, at an individual level, far worse than smoking, and life expectancy for those people who are alcohol dependent is significantly lower than it is even for smokers. Those who combine both habits of course are worst off of all.

What you might not have appreciated though is that taking regular, short breaks from the booze can dramatically alter your body's response. Giving your liver a break every week for a few days can have an extremely positive effect, and can also significantly reduce (if not eliminate) your chances of becoming physically dependent[vii]. And from the point of view of developing a "business" solution to this, that is good news indeed, because selling people on becoming "teetotal" didn't feel to me like a marketing challenge I wanted to take up.

So stopping being alcohol dependent does not mean giving up altogether, it just means managing to mix drinking days with non-drinking days in a sensible manner.

Smoking:

Although it's pretty hard to hide the fact you are a smoker, many people do. If you are a smoker, you need to accept you are going to have to stop if you want to live longer.

The latest ONS (Office for National Statistics) data from 2013 show that almost one in five adults in the UK still smoke[viii]. That number is coming down (it's actually halved since the mid 1970s), but it's still high, and represents around 11m people. Men are stuck at 22%, but the good news is rates of smoking amongst women are now down at 17%, down 2% on 2012.

And although there are folk who will have "the occasional smoke", social smokers only make up around 10% of this group (1.1m people), and still smoke on average 37 cigarettes a week, according to a study undertaken by

University College London – and are still putting themselves at increased risk of many smoking-related diseases[ix].

There's no adverse judgement here from me on smoking. I was a smoker myself, before I stopped in my mid-30s.

Obesity:

Almost two thirds of the adult population in the UK are either overweight or obese, defined by reference to their BMI (Body Mass Index) (Health & Safety Executive, HSE, data, 62.1%, 2013). Similar figures apply in the US, although some European countries do seem to have a better handle on this, with much lower figures.

BMI is a single number calculated by looking at both your height and weight to determine how thin or fat you are. It's a very imperfect measure, but the only one we really have to work with on a population-wide basis. Most people don't know what their BMI is, or that the BMI trigger for clinical obesity is a measure of 30. The average adult BMI is well over 27, which is comfortably into the "overweight" category, and if you look at the graph below you can see what BMI category you fall into. This graph uses a better, modified formula to work out your BMI than the standard version some people might be familiar with (there's more on this later in the book and you can work out your exact BMI using this formula on thelifeofrileybook.com website).

Being overweight (i.e. having a BMI between 25 and 30) does not appear at first sight to cause significant life expectancy issues[x], although the data is not altogether clear on this, and I explore the complexities of it all on the website. However, being overweight may cause more health problems in later life, and being obese (i.e. having a BMI over 30) definitely starts to become a problem from the perspective of longevity, and the more obese you are, the worse it seems to get, according to a major study by the NHS National Obesity Observatory[xi].

From reviewing all of the data, the lifestyle and age-related life-expectancy effects of obesity seem to be scalable, as you'd expect. And the NHS NOO study suggests it's roughly 1 year of lost life for every point over 30 on the BMI scale. So getting your weight down so your BMI is below 30 would appear to eliminate most, if not all, of the adverse life expectancy effects of being obese.

In the UK, many people are in self-denial about being overweight, with even those people technically measured as being clinically obese content to describe themselves as "comfortable with their weight". In fact, a recent study by Cancer Research UK reported in *The Times*[xii] found that 90% of obese people simply didn't recognise that about themselves, thinking they were just overweight, or even normal weight. This finding was backed up by the most recent HSE report on the topic[xiii].

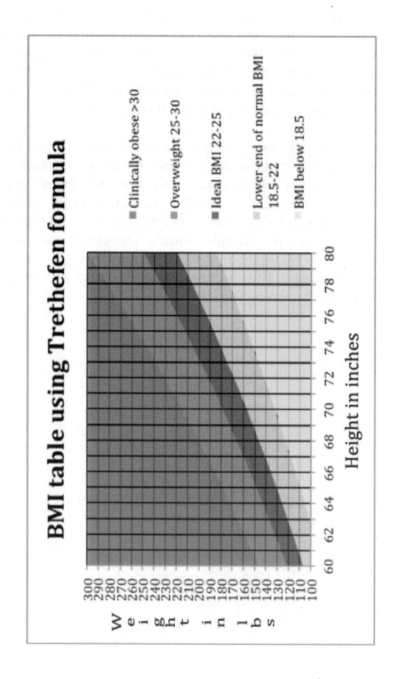

BMI table using Trethefen formula

Height in inches

- Clinically obese >30
- Overweight 25-30
- Ideal BMI 22-25
- Lower end of normal BMI 18.5-22
- BMI below 18.5

Media images don't help here, because they tend to show pictures of the most obese individuals when discussing the condition, so people see those pictures (love handles sticking out of too small T Shirts for example) and think "that's not me, so I can't be obese". It also doesn't help that the term obese is considered derogatory.

A report published in May 2015 by the European Association for the Study of Obesity (reported in *The Guardian* with the obligatory misleading picture) confirms this depressing fact about our continuing denial[xiv].

Again, I am not going to make any judgements about individuals here, and the reason is because in 2000, at the age of 40, I was clinically obese, with a BMI of 33 (6 years after I had stopped smoking). One recent large-scale study from Kings College in London put the chances of you successfully losing weight if you were an obese man at 1 in 210, and for women 1 in 124[xv].

Those are pretty tough odds, but I don't believe they need to be that high. I'm convinced anyone can make the dietary changes to move away from obesity – and far more simply than they might think.

Based on the numbers of people in each category of obesity, the average obese person has a BMI of around 35, thereby lopping between 4 and 5 years off his or her life (check out thelifeofrileybook.com for more details on this statistic). In addition of course, being obese brings with it lifestyle challenges, making later life more difficult in many respects (as of course do smoking and heavy drinking).

But losing that weight can be done.

Physical Inactivity:

Finally we are, as a nation, nowhere near as physically active as we should be.

Going back to business basics, an oft-used quote is "if you can't measure it, you can't manage it", and measuring fitness is challenging. It would normally require some scientific apparatus to check your heart rate or breathing effort when you are exposed to stressful activity such as walking uphill on a treadmill or cycling on a stationary bike. This is what you would expect to go through if you had a full-blown medical or expensive health check-up. Simpler measures do exist, such as how quickly you can walk a mile, or how many press-ups you can do, but they are awfully compromised by age, gender, race and pre-existing levels of activity, which all conspire to make a "one size fits all" measure of fitness hard to create.

For interest, your resting heart rate is about as good a measure as any[xvi], but you need to check it first thing, before you have sprung out of bed, and certainly before you have had that first coffee. Depending upon age and sex the average resting heart rate is in the low to mid 70s, so if yours is higher than that this might indicate a lack of fitness, and if it's lower, again it might indicate you are more physically active than most. Even with this one measure, resting heart rate, there is no single answer because of individual factors that might be at play. This is why directly measuring fitness in a simple manner is so difficult.

Given that directly measuring fitness is so difficult, the best proxy we have is measuring physical activity, because we know the two things are directly correlated. For simplicity, I will use both fitness and physical activity as shorthand terms in the book, but I am going to ask you to measure your physical activity as the key determinant of your fitness as we go forward.

Well over half of us claim to achieve government physical activity goals each week when asked, yet closer examination reveals far fewer of us are actually putting in that amount of effort.

In the official annual UK Government self-completed surveys for the HSE[xvii], in 2012 around two thirds of all men and over half of all women claimed to be physically active to the relevant guidelines (i.e. they do 150 minutes per week of moderate physical activity).

But these top-line "self-reported" estimates of physical activity are widely known to be flawed[xviii].

When more detailed analysis is undertaken, the real rate drops – dramatically – to around 20%. Only around one third of the actual level claimed.

A team at the University of Bristol looked at recent data from the Sport England "Active People Survey", and discovered from the respondents that *"nearly 80 per cent did not meet the minimum criteria of moderate exercise at least 12 times in a four-week period"*[xix].

Crikey – what a nation of fibbers we are.

I might have done the same fibbing myself during my 20s and 30s. I dabbled a bit in jogging in my early/mid 20s – round the park, two or three miles at a time. But I'm 6ft 5ins tall, so running is ruinously bad for me, and I was simply not very good, and not very fast. I swam a bit, but again, finding the time, and the pool, was not always easy. So I stopped exercising as my 20s drew to a close. And did absolutely nothing throughout my 30s. Hence the discovery, around my 40th birthday, that I was both clinically obese, and completely, utterly, chronically unfit.

I know I am not alone. Busy careers, late nights working, young families, or looking after elderly relatives all conspire to mean many adults in their 30s and 40s simply abandon physical exercise. And then never manage to pick it up again.

That was me, aged 40. Obese, and completely and utterly unfit.

The sedentary do not live as long, on average, as the physically active. But managing a couple of hours or so of physical exercise every week is easier than you imagine – and there is a lot of evidence that even a proportion of that goes a long, long way towards delivering the longevity benefits of the UK Government 150 minute target[xx]. In fact, in a recent study in Taiwan over a 12-year period, reported in *The Lancet*[xxi], even people who only exercised for 90 minutes a week had a life expectancy 3 years longer than those who were inactive. Other studies have shown even greater gains for just slightly more effort.

And lycra need not be involved at all. We're going to set out a physical activity plan in a couple of chapters. I think you'll be pleased at its simplicity.

So, I'm not talking about asking you to transform yourself into an ultra-fit triathlete here. But if the lifestyle changes you make can include…

Stopping smoking cigarettes;

Not drinking for a few days every week;

Losing enough weight not to be considered obese; and

Getting out of the house or from behind your desk for 30 minutes, 4 times a week to go for moderate exercise

… you will be amazed at how that change can potentially transform both your life expectancy prospects and the quality of your later years. And measuring how well you are doing on these changes is pretty easy to do.

And this change can happen at any time of life, with the beneficial effects starting almost immediately.

Realistically though, if you are already in your 60s and want to shift from being a heavy-drinking, obese, sedentary smoker into a lean, non-smoking moderate drinking fitness fanatic (virtually) overnight you might not expect to get all of the life-expectancy enhancing benefits of a 30 year-old doing the same thing, but the positive effects will start from the day you make the change.

I doubt there are many people reading this book who are at risk from all four horsemen, so the likelihood is you probably only need to change one or two aspects of your lifestyle. You will need to crack all four lifestyle changes if you can – doing just three still leaves you at risk from the fourth horseman and his scythe. I appreciate too that every single change might be a challenge, as changing habits is difficult, so the plan itself is staged, so as not to look too daunting to begin with.

And why should you change habits – what's in it for you?

Well I would say three things stand out.

First – the quantitative benefit. You should, on average live longer – possibly by a decade or more. And that's extra 'good life". We are all likely to face some "inconvenience" in our last few years on earth – but that's true whether we are going to pass on aged 70 or 90 – and it's the extra years of good health that count. So you get more time for you to enjoy.

Second – the qualitative benefit. Following *The Life of Riley* habits should mean better health in those later years, so not only is the quantity of life improved – so is the quality. Thus allowing you to do more of the things you've always dreamed of – not necessarily bungee jumping in New Zealand – but if that's what floats your boat then go for it. Travel is probably the top "bucket list" thing for most of us – whether its simply to marvel at the sights you've always wanted to see, explore and be adventurous, or simply to visit friends and relatives – being fit enough to travel is therefore a key part of ticking off those bucket list dreams.

Third – the emotional benefit. It gives others more time with you. Here I am specifically thinking of the next generation, and the one after that. There is no more powerful human urge than the desire to see our children do well, and then in turn enjoy nurturing our grand-children, and possibly beyond. I think you can add an extra generation to those you can love by living longer.

I'll capture all of these benefits (and some more we'll discover later) in a summary at the end of the book, but I hope for now they are enough for you to keep reading.

In order to make a change, you have to acknowledge that you need to, so I would ask you to make an honest assessment as to whether any of these poorer lifestyle choices applies to you, and more importantly, if you want to do something about it.

I then hope in the next few chapters to both give you a compelling reason why you should make a change, and some easy ways to make a difference.

And *The Life of Riley* habits pull all of those changes into one simple routine.

Chapter 3

"Ordinary average guy"

Ordinary average guy – Joe Walsh

I'm a numbers geek.

I've always been very comfortable with numbers, and that has helped me lots in my career. I did my first degree at Loughborough (Seb Coe was a contemporary, along with loads of other now-famous athletes – who of course didn't have much time for us "numbers guys"!) My degree was in Computer Studies, but in those days (the 1970s) computing degrees were run out of maths departments. So for a Computer Studies degree, boy did we do a lot of maths. Including a lot of statistics. I loved it.

Later, I did an MBA at Columbia Business School in New York. Because I'd been out of University for six years by then, they made me redo a bunch of maths as an entrance test – including stats again. So I had to relearn it all. Loved it again.

So much so, the news editors who have worked with me over the years will testify to a man (and woman) about my annoyance when we get stats and number stories wrong in our news bulletins. Some of the time it's unscrupulous PR agencies trying to pull the wool over journalists' eyes regarding a product they are selling – or more frequently politicians trying to spin some scheme or other. It makes my blood boil.

Stick with me here, because I'm going to do the numbers so you don't have to. I've explained it all on thelifeofrileybook.com if you really are interested, but for everyone else the top line findings are the important bit, which I will explain below. I know for most people their eyes glaze over if someone even mentions maths, so let me summarise here what the data says.

The oft-quoted average (mean) life expectancy in the UK is 79 (77 for men, 81 for women[xxii]). However, this number suffers from three flaws.

First, it includes the tragic deaths of babies, infants and young people – virtually none of whom are dying from the sort of lifestyle related illnesses we are discussing in this book. Just looking at adult life expectancy (people over the age of 30 seems a sensible starting point) would therefore considerably increase average figures.

Second, the published numbers fail to include all the people who are now expected to live beyond 100, despite more of them being around than ever before, and their longevity being due to a combination of good genes and more importantly living a healthy lifestyle (good genes won't save you from a bad lifestyle). Adding these people in will boost the numbers too.

Finally, the 79 number is the arithmetic average (mean) which means it is dragged down by the sheer numbers of folk dying really early (like my friends) in their 50s and 60s. Using a different average (the median, or "mid-point" measure) is much better for this type of analysis[xxiii].

If instead therefore, we look at the "adult" average, i.e. only focussing on people who live to at least 30, and include our expected over 100 year old veterans, and take the median average (the 50/50 halfway point) rather than mean (the arithmetic average), then average life expectancy for adults living in the UK today increases to 84 (82 for men and 86 for women).

So forget living to 79, as an adult alive today you have a 50:50 chance of living to 84. In the graph below, the first "white" bar is the 0-100 mean, the second "white" bar is the 30-100 median. That's quite some gap between what we think, and what the data actually says.

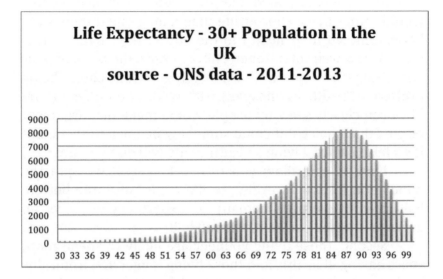

Now that's probably shocked you. It might even have frightened you if you are worried about finances and living comfortably etc. And I'd agree with you that living longer isn't always all good news.

In fact, recent estimates suggest that while 84 is a very useful guide to median (50/50) adult life expectancy, once you get to 65 you might only expect 10 years or so of healthy life, followed by, on average, up to the last 8 years of life lived in varying degrees of ill-health, according to data from the Kings Fund[xxiv]. Now ill-health is a broad term, which could cover a range of challenges from simply having to take a pill or two every day, through to significant disease or infirmity. Those of us in our 40s and 50s will be facing this now of course, having to look after aged parents and other relatives.

This isn't great, and it's one reason why, when I've been talking to people about this book, and the concept of *The Life of Riley* habits, one recurring theme crops up, which is the argument "I don't want to live another five or six years if it's going to be in a care home or in and out of hospital". In fact, a recent study said that, if given the choice, people would rather live a shorter life than a long one if they could be guaranteed their health to the end of their lives[xxv]. This study was a well-intentioned effort to raise the issue of poor end-of-life care – one well worth doing. But the choice being proffered (health vs. lifespan) isn't what is on offer in real life. I can clearly see why people would make that argument or pick that choice if it could somehow be open to them. But it's a false choice. Living a healthier life will do two things.

First, it will allow you to live longer. If we split the population in two according to life expectancy, the bottom half have an average (median) life expectancy of 75, vs. an average (median) of 90 for the top half.

Second, those dying younger are likely to spend more years having ill health, and those living longer are, ironically, likely to spend fewer years in ill-health. Let's take that 8 year average estimate for years of ill health supplied by the Kings Fund and assume those in the bottom half are actually suffering a little more ill health, say 10 years, and those in the top half a little less, say 6 years.

This means the bottom half of the population start getting ill on average aged 65, whilst the top half don't reach that state until 84.

So the gap in terms of healthy life is almost 20 years between the top half and the bottom half, if my 10 and 6 is right (actual data splitting healthy life vs. life expectancy is pretty sketchy unfortunately but I'm pretty confident from all the data that many of those folk who get into their 80s and beyond are pretty sprightly in the main). That's potentially two decades of extra, enjoyable life, and a lot less of any inconvenience (and I suspect less intensive inconvenience to boot).

Now of course socio-economic factors such as poverty and poor living conditions affect whether or not people end up in the bottom or top half of life expectancy (and I'll talk about these factors in more detail in chapter 13), but making lifestyle changes can dramatically change the outcomes for you as an individual, no matter what your socio-economic circumstances.

And if you follow the habits I describe later, I think you can do a lot better than just getting into the "top half" of that table. In the next chapter I want to introduce you to the five Tribes.

Chapter 4

"Song for the Tribes"

Song for the tribes – Simple Minds

This is where it gets interesting. Because life expectancy seems to depend in large part on which Tribe you belong to. And the evidence shows we rather neatly divide into five Tribes – heavy/frequent drinkers (Tribe 1); sober smokers (Tribe 2); the clinically obese (Tribe 3), the sedentary (Tribe 4); and the live longers (Tribe 5). If you think you might fit into more than one Tribe, go with the lower number.

In a business setting, if we had identified Tribes 1-4 as our target markets, and were developing a product that would attract them and move them to Tribe 5, we would at this point be planning what is known as "qual/quant" research. Basically this means performing a large research project with a balanced cross-section of each group to understand what's going on in their lives, followed by some smaller scale focus groups, to talk to them on an individual level – possibly testing some initial marketing ideas.

Luckily for me, we don't need to do that here. Science has very kindly supplied us with more research than you could shake a stick at. In fact probably too much (and some of course contradictory), and I am therefore only going to share with you what appear to me to be the key bits of data about each Tribe.

But the data does start to get a little spread out here. When death certificates are issued, age and gender is recorded, along with cause of death. But not lifestyle choices. Death certificates don't say, "he was a smoker"; "she never touched a drop in her life"; "he was obese"; "she ran a marathon every month"; "he was a real couch potato".

Perhaps they should – and there are some people asking for smoking behaviour at least to be recorded. But it isn't now, and neither are any of those other lifestyle factors. So the data is not as comprehensive as we'd like. But here's what we do know, or can calculate using the available data and a bit of maths.

In the analysis below I need to make a couple of rules clear.

First, you can only be in one Tribe.

Second, I'm afraid it's the one that will deliver the worst outcome for you (Tribe 1 is the worst, then Tribe 2 etc.). So if you are both a heavy/frequent drinker and clinically obese, I'd put you in Tribe 1. If you are both sedentary and a smoker, you are in Tribe 2. Only if you can avoid being in all of the first 4 Tribes do you get to be in the live longer Tribe, Tribe 5.

Tribe 1:

The heavy/frequent drinkers.

I described the nature of heavy/frequent drinking in chapter 2. What about the size of the problem?

Data collated by the UK Health and Social Care Information Centre (NHSCIC) from 2007 shows that up to 25% of all adults are consuming "hazardous" amounts of alcohol on a regular basis[xxvi]. This is the precursor level to "harmful drinking", which is itself the stage before becoming "alcohol-dependent". The research estimates that around 9% of men and 4% of women show some signs of being alcohol dependent[xxvii].

I must say that from a practical perspective, these labels are unhelpful. To have three levels of problem drinking, namely "hazardous"; "harmful" and "alcohol dependent" is bad enough, but to label the two less damaging levels as "hazardous" and "harmful" seems perverse – they sound much worse than simply being dependent. And would you be able to tell which of "hazardous" and "harmful" was the less severe, unless I'd already told you?

I prefer to simply refer to those of us who drink too much as heavy/frequent drinkers, as I think the word "dependent" can allow some people to consider themselves not at risk if they do not feel addicted in any sense. I'm also not convinced those of us sitting quietly at home getting a bit sloshed every evening would instinctively consider that "hazardous" or "harmful" behaviour. We probably think "hazardous" is somehow related to young men and women falling down drunk late at night in risky situations. That probably is hazardous of course – but so too potentially is the effect on our livers of all that regular tipsiness.

We can get in an awful tangle over drinking in the UK. A recent, survey published by *The British Medical Journal* (which was widely publicised in the press, and then nicely skewered in his blog by Christopher Snowden[xxviii]), reported on the "epidemic' of drinking occurring in wealthier/healthier over 50s. The use of the word epidemic was unhelpful to begin with, and the study didn't actually pinpoint quite what was so terrible about otherwise healthy middle-class people sitting at home having a couple of glasses of wine each evening.

However, we mustn't dismiss all of this as simply "nanny state nagging", because there's clearly a spectrum here. Couples splitting one bottle of wine between them three nights a week would almost certainly fit into the category of "moderate drinkers". Couples who have most of a couple of bottles over dinner, seven nights a week, are clearly well on the way to being "heavy/frequent drinkers".

Heavy/frequent drinking is far more widespread and problematic for public health than I think we like to admit, and we are as a nation in denial about how much we drink. The data for actual amounts of alcohol sold are hugely different to those that are implied when we tell researchers how much we consume. A recent widely reported study from Liverpool's John Moores University[xxix] reckons there are a missing 12 million bottles of wine drunk every week in the UK that we didn't mention to the researchers. Wine though only accounts for around one third of all alcoholic consumption in the UK, and I don't imagine wine drinkers are any more or less truthful than anyone else. So if you therefore add in the missing pints and spirits I also imagine aren't being properly reported, that adds up to a lot of booze.

Dr Mark Porter wrote a very interesting article in *The Times*[xxx] (to which I will return) that estimated some two million Brits have a serious drink problem. That's a smaller number than the NHSCIC data above, at about 4% of the adult population, but ties in very well to a more substantial German study on drinking which ran from 1996 to 2010 and which I have used as the base for my own modelling[xxxi] (Germany and the UK have almost identical levels of per capita alcohol consumption). This study was actually looking at whether alcohol treatment centres have any effect – and sadly they didn't appear to be of much benefit – but the research threw up some fascinating background data that I've used.

This study suggested that alcohol-dependent drinkers make up around 6% of the male population and around 1.5% of the female population – so around 4% overall, in line with Dr Porter's estimate. The study also suggested that average (mean) life expectancy for these heavy/frequent drinkers was just 58 for men and 60 for women. This age correlates closely to the figures recorded by the UK Government on specific alcohol-related deaths in the UK, where the average (mean) age is 61 for men and 60 for women (although specifically alcohol-related recorded deaths are a very small number it should be said, and those people who are heavy/frequent drinkers are dying from a range of conditions, which are mainly not recorded as being alcohol-specific).

I am going to use the German 6% for men and 1.5% for women figures going forward as it is the most robustly researched I can find, and is perhaps a bit more prudent than the NHS 9%/4% figures I started with.

By the way, a lot of this Tribe also smoke – four out of five according to the German study – much, much higher than in the population as a whole (the prevalence of smoking amongst heavy drinkers is an entire field of scientific study). That double effect of both smoking and heavy/frequent drinking for nearly all of those in Tribe 1 is why their average life expectancy numbers are so low.

I don't think 4% is an "epidemic" by any stretch of the imagination, but it is a significant figure, especially for men, where 6% equates to around 1 man in every 15. You only need to look around any large office containing, say, 100 people split equally between men and women to reckon on 3 or 4 of the men and 1 of the women being in the heavy/frequent drinker category. We should therefore take it seriously.

Tribe 2:

Should technically be defined as "smokers who either only drink moderately, or abstain altogether". It's probably easier though to use the shorthand of "sober smokers" to describe them, even though they may drink at sensible levels.

We know from the UK Government data in 2013 I quoted earlier that 22% of men and 17% of women smoke. Out of that overall group, we need to take out those smokers who are also heavy drinkers (and who we have therefore already counted in Tribe 1). Once we've done that, Tribe 2, the "sober smokers", is 17% of all adult men, and 16% of all adult women.

We often hear quoted the statistic that smokers live around a decade less than non-smokers. Using the average (median) whole-population adult (30+) life expectancy of 84 (82 for men, 86 for women) I quoted earlier as the base, this implies smokers in general (i.e. both sober and drinkers) have a median life expectancy of around 74 if they are men, and 77 if they are women (as non-smokers will be living a little longer than the adult whole population median). This estimate is backed up by recent research on very large samples (in the hundreds of thousands) by the USA Centers for Disease Control and Prevention[xxxii], and the Australian National University[xxxiii]. Professor Emily Banks, who ran the Australian study, confirmed this to me when we spoke, telling me her data suggested almost half (45%) of all smokers (men and women) had already died by 75, which was the age at which her study stopped.

Interestingly though, if you remove the drinker/smokers, whom we already accounted for in Tribe 1, the sober smokers in Tribe 2 have an average (mean) age of death of 79 for both sexes. That's possibly higher than you might expect, but is still 5 years younger than the overall adult average life expectancy of 84, and within that, just comparing them to non-smokers will push the margin out to 6-7 years.

Tribe 3:

As I reported earlier, obese people represent around a quarter (25%) of the UK adult population. These are people with a BMI greater than 30.

According to the data, just under one in five of them also smoke[xxxiv], in line with the general population, so we have already accounted for these folk in Tribe 2 (or even in Tribe 1 if they are also heavy/frequent drinkers).

Therefore the non-smoking obese represent around 20% of the UK population (slightly more men than women), and are my Tribe 3. On balance, the men are also slightly heavier within this category, certainly in the top end category of morbid obesity (a BMI of 40+).

On average, according to UK data, obese people in general live between 4 and 5 years less than those who are not obese (see thelifeofrileybook.com for these statistics) – with average (mean) life expectancy at 79 for men, and 82 for women. However, those people who are both obese and smoke will be dragging this average down to a degree, so after we have adjusted for the obese smokers who are in Tribe 2 by stripping them out of these calculations, the average (mean) life expectancy for Tribe 3 (non-smoking obese) is just over 80 for men, and just under 84 for women.

So if being obese is your only health issue (i.e. you don't drink and don't smoke) its effect on your longevity is not quite as dramatic as the newspaper headlines make out – but it will still place you in the bottom half of the population as far as life expectancy is concerned, and of course expose you to increased health issues as you get older.

Between them, Tribes 1, 2 and 3 make up around 40% of the total UK population, and all of them have a predicted average life expectancy that falls short of their 84th birthday – in many cases well short.

As 84 is the overall average life expectancy for the adult population at large, that's exactly what we'd expect.

For reference, 44% of men are in Tribes 1-3, vs. only 36% of women. I won't bore you with the maths here, but this difference on its own explains about half of overall life expectancy differences between the sexes.

So we are left with the 60% who are either in Tribe 4 (the sedentary) or the live longers in Tribe 5.

Tribe 4:

The sedentary, are interesting.

The UK Government definition of being fit is taking part in moderate to intense physical activity for 150 minutes a week (i.e. half an hour, five days a week), or intense activity for 75 minutes a week. And it does seem to be the case that it's physical activity that is important here. You can of course feel "fit and well" of course for much of your life without doing anything remotely "exercise" based – which might be a problem, from a longevity perspective.

According to that data from the University of Bristol study that I referred to earlier[xix], only around 20% of UK adults complete enough regular exercise (i.e. 3 times a week over a month) to qualify as fit. The data seems to split pretty evenly between men and women – although there are much bigger differences by ethnicity, with those of African, Caribbean or Asian descent doing worse, and also big splits by income, with better off folk doing better from an exercise perspective. None of those splits is surprising – but as far as exercise is concerned, nothing here is written in stone – your destiny shouldn't be decided by your race, or social background, or wealth.

This of course is also true for smoking, heavy/frequent drinking and obesity – you are the master of your own fate in all of these things.

I am going to assume for simplicity's sake that no one in Tribes 1, 2 or 3 is particularly physically active. In reality I know this isn't completely true, as some obese people are trying to lose weight via exercise (which on its own doesn't really work), and others are managing to be both heavy drinkers and physically active (I know because I did this for more than a decade), but from a mathematical modelling perspective it makes life easier.

If this is the case, then the remaining 60% of the population must be split pretty much two thirds sedentary, one third physically active.

I've assumed roughly even parity between men and women here. Although the Active People Survey[xxxv] suggests slightly more men do some sport (40% of men vs. 30% of women do at least one 30 minute burst of exercise a week), there isn't any compelling data on gender splits in the 20% who are keeping regularly active.

So if 40% of the population are in Tribes 1, 2 or 3, and of the remainder only 20% are regularly physically active, then the sedentary must account for almost 40% of the population as a whole. Tribe 4 therefore, the sedentary, is the biggest Tribe of all.

How much is exercise worth though, in terms of increased life expectancy? Harvard University has conducted an overarching study of all of the exercise-related research, and their conclusions are impressive[xxxvi]. Just two hours a week of moderate physical activity (actually below UK government guidelines) should add three years or longer to your life, compared to doing no exercise at all. If you go the whole hog and really embrace physical fitness, you can add up to four and a half years.

For the purposes of my modelling, I've taken three and a half years as a typical life expectancy extension for a physically active person. This number is backed up by other meta-analyses of exercise data[xxxvii].

That means the Tribe 4 sedentary men have an average (mean) life expectancy of 86, and for Tribe 4 sedentary women it's 88.

Pulling this all together, how does that add up in terms of life expectancy by Tribe?

Here's what it looks like by Tribe, assuming 100,000 people are being measured overall (which is what the ONS data does).

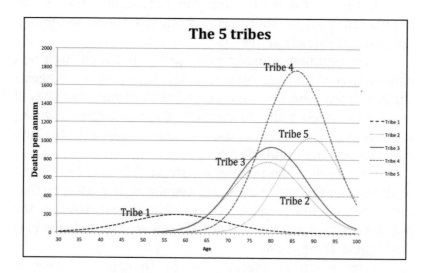

And if you put all of these Tribes together, the overall picture from the model looks like this (this is just the male version)

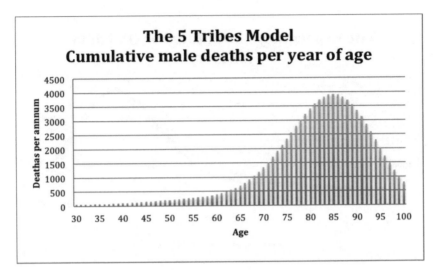

That looks remarkably like the official data from the ONS

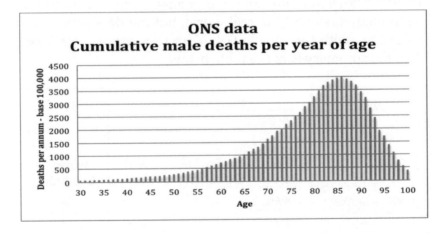

And in fact, if you put them side by side, this is what it looks like:

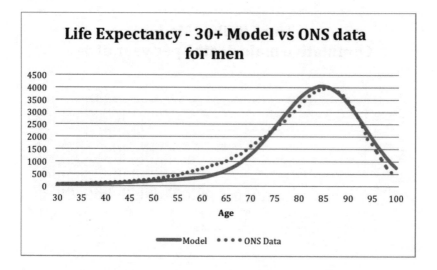

I've explained the detailed modelling on thelifeofrileybook.com, and the model is by its nature a simplified version of the real world, but the data suggests it correlates with the official ONS data to a remarkable 99%. And the summary is in the table below:

	Men		Women	
	% of Popln	Median Life Expectancy	% of Popln	Median Life Expectancy
Tribe 1 – drinkers	5.8%	58	1.5%	60
Tribe 2 – smokers	17.4%	79	15.8%	79
Tribe 3 – obese	20.8%	80	19.0%	84
Tribe 4 – sedentary	36.0%	86	43.7%	88
Tribe 5	20.0%	89	20.0%	91

Tribe 5:

And the big news is this.

All of the data points in one direction.

If you can get into Tribe 5 – the live longers – your median life expectancy is 89 for men and 91 for women.

I think this is simply incredible.

It's over a decade older than the oft-quoted 79 we've been talking about so far in this book, and it's a whopping 15 years more than the average (median) for everyone in Tribes 1-3.

From a sales and marketing perspective, living until you are around 90 is a pretty good number to use as the key benefit of the plan – an increase of up to 15 years compared to the 3 poorest lifestyle choices, and probably much longer in terms of "healthy life" – probably a couple of decades.

By the way, I'm not the first person to have estimated the negative and positive effects of different lifestyle habits on life expectancy. In fact, Professor David Spiegelhalter from Cambridge University has posted an interesting paper on "effective age", which captures many of the same ideas and comes to quite similar conclusions[xxxviii].

Chapter 5

"Time takes a cigarette"

Rock'n'Roll Suicide – David Bowie

Stopping smoking is hard.

I know. I was a smoker.

So before we get to *The Life of Riley* habits, we need to discuss smoking, and how you can stop. Because it can be done – and perhaps more easily than you might think. (If you aren't a smoker, you can skip this chapter if you want.)

I need to be upfront with you here. I don't have a magic, easy-to-follow plan for stopping smoking, and it isn't strictly part of *The Life of Riley* habits. All I can do is give you a bit of my history, talk through what seems to work (and not work) and point you in the direction of some resources that might help you.

My mum and dad were both smokers, although my dad gave up in the 1960s when he was about 35, after a particularly bad bout of pneumonia. I think he was actually at death's door, but it wasn't talked about in the house. Anyway, he recovered, but never smoked again – although the desire never left him. If I lit up using a match near him he used to tell me the smell of the burning sulphur was enough to trigger the memories of his smoking days. He had been quite physically active too in his youth, cycling everywhere, and doing his national service. He was still an active, manual type of guy, fixing cars both for work and in his spare time.

He contracted bowel cancer in his late 50s, and of course I've no idea if it was in any way related to his smoking. He had a large bowel resection, which gave him a few extra years, but the cancer came back elsewhere, and he died in his early 60s when I was in my mid 30s. Sadly he only knew his two grand-daughters as little girls, and never got to meet his grand-son, who was born shortly after he had died.

And I think that is one of the reasons I wanted to do this analysis and write this book – to try and encourage people to change their lifestyles if they can, so they can live longer and do more – and critically for most people that includes seeing their families grow. And in particular seeing grandchildren grow up. If your grandchildren are born when you are in your 60s, and you don't live beyond your 70s, you will miss a great deal of them growing up – and the joy that can bring.

My mum lasted longer than my dad, despite smoking her entre adult life. She just could not be persuaded to give up cigarettes, no matter how hard I tried in later life, after I had stopped myself.

She had grown up in Dublin in the 40s and 50s, and had worked for a time at Players, one of the big cigarette companies of that era, who had a factory just a mile or so down the road from where the Kinsellas lived in Inchicore. Everyone smoked in Ireland (and drank too of course!) and my mum was no exception.

It is no real surprise therefore that I, as the working class child of two smokers in 1970s Manchester, started smoking myself in my teenage years.

I smoked initially until my mid-twenties, and stopped for a while, as my broadcasting life took off (I suspect I did realise ruining my throat was not a good career move for someone who used their voice every day). I then left England in 1986, as I was fortunate enough to gain entrance to Columbia Business School in New York.

I may have been introduced to some unusual cigarettes while there. And unlike Bill Clinton, from time to time I did inhale! Next thing you know, I'm back on the cigarettes. (I should just say I did not spend two years in a drug-induced stupor – doing my MBA was actually the hardest, but most intellectually rewarding time of my life).

When I returned to the UK in 1988, I decided that as an aspiring radio businessman I needed to move on from cigarettes, so took up smoking cigars instead. What a mistake that was. Three packs of Hamlet a day was literally burning my money away, and was probably worse for my throat than the cigarettes I used to smoke.

I stuck with the cigars until I was 33.

I gave up on June 4th 1993, my 34th birthday. Jean, my wife, bought me Alan Carr's *Easy way to stop smoking*, which I'm glad to see is still in print. Not to be confused with chat show host Alan Carr, this Alan Carr was a former smoker (100 a day for 33 years) who had created a method of quitting, which he ran both in group sessions, and via a series of books.

I read the book over the course of a day, and stopped instantly. I've never picked up a cigarette or cigar since. Nor will I ever do so again. I won't tell you what the book talks about, but it was a simple notion, which worked perfectly for me.

Sadly Alan's previous history of smoking caught up with him, and he died of lung cancer in 2006 aged 72 – but not before helping many tens (if not hundreds) of thousands of people to stop smoking. Good on him – I personally am forever in his debt.

The reason I stopped on my 34th birthday was that Jean was about to give birth to our first daughter, Alexandra, a month or so later, and I didn't want her to be living in a house full of smoke – or be a dad who wasn't there for her when she grew up because I had inadvertently killed myself with cigarettes or cigars.

But as you will know if you are a smoker, the willingness and motivation can be there – but if the method doesn't work, you are still going to end up back on the cigs.

The great news is that we know so much more about

the psychology and physiology of smoking now that it really is possible to tailor a method to you as an individual that works. ·

Alan's book is essentially a way of getting you to change your worldview, and is certainly a first port of call I would recommend for someone who is prepared to think clearly about his or her habit and how they might change.

Alan's approach was also designed to be used as part of a group "hypnotherapy" approach, and I know of people for whom that has worked – although I suspect if I had done it while under hypnotherapy, I could imagine convincing myself later that it was "wearing off", so for me reading the book, stone-cold sober, was a better approach.

In the NHS/government world of smoking cessation there are "good" ways to quit, and "bad" ways to quit. For me, there are only ways that work, and ways that don't. And for every individual, he or she might need to try both the orthodox and unorthodox in order to succeed.

When I stopped smoking, patches hadn't been invented. Nor had gum. Certainly e-cigs were nowhere to be seen. There are now drugs too, which need a doctor's prescription of course, but again these are fairly recent additions to the arsenal of those wanting to stop.

I don't have a magic cure. But I know that this combination of self-help books; hypnotherapy; patches; gum; nasal sprays & lozenges; drugs; and now e-cigs is helping hundreds of thousands of people each year stop in the UK. And smoking rates have halved since the mid-70s when I first started, so it can be done.

Ranking the various methods, I would go in the following order:

1. Try just stopping if you feel you have the will power. I suspect that's where Alan's book (and/or hypnotherapy comes in) for people who probably think they can go cold-turkey, but just need a bit of mental help to get them going.

2. If that doesn't work, try the gum, or patches, or spray. It's the nicotine to which you are addicted, so breaking the addiction from the mechanistic smoking activity is a first, key step. If you can then reduce the nicotine dosage over time via patches, gum etc. you stand a good chance of cracking it.
3. If that doesn't work, go see your doctor and ask for some prescribed medication. Good drugs, with quite high success rates, do exist and your doctor will either know of them him/herself, or can point you in the right NHS direction. But they'll probably want to know you've tried and failed with the other methods before prescribing you drugs – hence this is point three on the list.
4. Finally, if you physically can't stop, try vaping. The new e-cigarette availability does appear to be leading to potentially faster rates of decline in actual cigarette smoking according to recent studies. There are of course questions about people continuing to consume something that is giving them a dose of a highly addictive (and potentially lethal) drug in the form of nicotine. But nicotine is the drug smokers are craving – and it's the smoke, not the nicotine, which is killing people.

My only worry with vaping is that you are not breaking the physical "cigarette in the hand" mental connection and you are therefore substituting one dependency for another. But, it's a dependency without the cigarette smoke, which, just to repeat, is what is actually killing smokers.

There are concerns about some of the other chemicals in the vaping mixture itself, but the consensus is that, although they may be harmful, they are not in the same league as tobacco smoke from the perspective of lung damage. Various estimates suggest they are 90% to 95% safer than cigarettes.

And the good news is recent research suggests that

vapers can go on to quit.

Ann McNeill, who conducted a recent study for Kings College into vaping[xxxix] was quoted in *The Times* as saying *"We're a little bit tired with people saying 'E-cigarettes are a bad thing, let's take them off the market'. It's not going to happen. E-cigarettes are here and research is pointing in the direction of them being helpful."*

Her research showed that, of the 1,500 smokers she tracked, 65% of those that used e-cigarettes every day had tried to fully quit – a much higher percentage than ordinary smokers at just 44%. Daily vapers were also twice as likely to halve their overall cigarette intake as non-vapers.

This research backed up previous studies in both the UK and New Zealand, which also showed vaping helped smokers quit.

Some other research claims vaping is no better than gum or patches for quitting, but even if it leads to a reduction, or cessation, of tobacco smoking in favour of pure vaping, that must be overall a beneficial outcome.

There is a concern amongst policy-makers that teens are picking up on the vaping habit (there's certainly some evidence from the US[xl]) but even this data is unclear, and vaping might be helping to stop many young people getting hooked on cigarettes in the first place.

However, the last word on vaping should probably go to The Royal College of Physicians, who published this statement on their website in March 2014 :

"...The main benefit of e-cigarettes is that they provide inhalable nicotine in a formulation that mimics the behavioural components of smoking but has relatively little risk... Switching completely from tobacco to e-cigarettes achieves much the same in health terms as does quitting smoking and all nicotine use completely. Furthermore... risks associated with passive exposure to e-cigarette vapour are far less than those associated with passive exposure to tobacco smoke..."

If only all professional bodies would follow suit and give advice with such clarity.

Let me finish by giving you one method of quitting that has been researched and has a better than 50% chance of working for you. What could this miracle technique be?

Well, it's an idea borrowed from the field of applied economics, and is called loss aversion. This refers to people's tendency to strongly prefer avoiding losses to acquiring gains.

This was shown to be really useful in helping people to quit, in an ingenious experiment conducted by scientists and reported in *The New England Journal of Medicine*[xli]. The smokers were offered four randomised methods of help or reward for quitting, including individual support or group support, or two types of cash rewards. The cash rewards beat support hands down in terms of effectiveness. However the two types of cash reward were subtly different. In one, smokers were simply offered an $800 reward to quit for 6 months. In the other, they were offered $650 in 6 months, but also had to place a $150 deposit down, which would be lost if they hadn't quit, or returned to them along with the $650 if they had quit.

Almost 90% of those offered the straight cash chose to participate (they had nothing to lose of course). Only 14% of those offered the "deposit + reward" programme agreed to participate. I suppose that's to be expected, with folk thinking at the outset they might lose their money. However, for those 14% that did, the potential "loss" of their deposit worked far better than simply offering a cash reward, with no loss if unsuccessful.

More than half of the deposit quitters had succeeded 6 months in, vs. only 17% of the straightforward cash offer quitters. So a little upfront investment paid off big time in terms of the chances of success in stopping.

There's a business parallel here. Most companies (and certainly Private Equity houses) expect their senior executives to have "skin in the game". They expect the people they are backing to run a business to have put some of their own personal wealth at risk too. I can assure you the loss aversion principal works for these executives, as they are then highly focussed on delivering returns – and I was one so I should know!

And it could work for you, by forcing you to make an investment in your own healthy future – buying a 50/50 chance of succeeding at stopping smoking (with all of the benefits) seems a pretty good return on, say, a £100 investment.

So if you really want to stop, give your partner, or parent, or other close relative £100 on the day you quit, with the deal they have to give it back to you, with another £100 (or more if you can persuade them), if you are still off the cigarettes 6 months later. You can vary the amounts as you see fit but I think you can see the picture of how loss aversion can work. You'll need to do this with someone who themselves has a vested interest in you stopping, and is therefore prepared to pay you the additional sum after six months – but you must have people in your life who want you to stop – so they are the ones to target. Make it a real wager though – with the money genuinely at risk.

The great news about quitting cigarettes is how much you can recover if you stop. The data shows that our bodies have remarkable powers of healing, such that 23 years after quitting, I have the lungs of a 40 year old (according to my latest medical), even though I am now 56.

According to a recent large scale Cancer Research UK study into women smokers and ex-smokers, "... Stopping before age 40 (and preferably well before age 40) avoids more than 90% of the excess mortality caused by continuing smoking; stopping before age 30 years avoids more than 97% of it[xlii]".

Stats for men are very similar. So you are getting 9 out of your 10 lost years back if you quit before you are 40.

Another US study found that smokers who quit in their mid-40s to mid-50s gained about six years. Those who quit later than this, but before age 65, gained up to four additional years[xliii]. It really is never too late to stop.

If you haven't stopped smoking yet, I'd urge you to find a bookmark, finish this chapter, and then attempt to stop. And if you don't succeed, attempt it again, with a different approach (some researchers reckon it might take up to seven attempts[xliv]). And keep attempting it until you succeed. None of the rest of this book will be of as much use to you if you are still smoking.

And, according to much scientific evidence (although again there is some debate), our reserves of willpower are limited.

Following *The Life of Riley* habits requires some willpower, at least initially. And I'd argue strongly most of us would not have sufficient willpower to both stop smoking, and start a new lifestyle plan at the same time. (If you are interested in willpower, there is a great book by Roy Baumeister, simply called "Willpower" which delves into this fascinating topic in great detail.)

Dying early, your body riddled with disease, missing out on the lives of your kids and grandkids. This is something you needn't fear if you can release the grip this habit has on you.

So let's deal with the smoking first. And stop.

Chapter 6

"For the Life of Riley"

The Life of Riley – Lightning Seeds

I'm going to work on the assumption you have stopped smoking (or more healthily never started, or at a pinch are purely vaping). If not, please go back and re-think the evidence in chapter 5. *The Life of Riley* habits simply won't work anywhere nearly as well if you are still smoking (although clearly they will be beneficial in other ways).

So here is the business proposition. *The Life of Riley* habits address all the other lifestyle issues you need to resolve in order to reduce ill-health and extend your life expectancy, in one, simple, five point structure that is easy to remember and straightforward to follow, for the rest of your life. The benefits are tangible and significant.

I'm assuming here that you want some help. If you are already a moderate drinker, who is not significantly overweight and takes physical activity seriously, you are probably already in Tribe 5. Well done. You can pick and choose from the habits as you see fit if you spot something you think is a good idea.

If you aren't yet in Tribe 5 (and if you're not sure, you probably aren't) then *The Life of Riley* habits are for you. And ideally you should follow them all, not just cherry-pick. The plan as a whole is designed to be followed as a cohesive whole.

It's worth saying here that the overall plan:

- Is not simply a diet;
- Is not primarily an exercise programme;

- Is not a self-help regime;
- Is not Alcoholics Anonymous.

It's just sticking to five habits on a regular basis, four days a week.

And these habits are based on the best scientific evidence I can find – not gut-feel or pseudo-scientific mumbo-jumbo based on things like blood groups or acid/alkaline balance, detoxing, juicing etc.

My objective here is to get you into Tribe 5, the live longers, and my strategy is to create a plan that is simple to follow.

None of the habits I am about to tell you are, in isolation, at all difficult to pick up.

Each of them is relatively modest. You might even think to the point of being banal. But that is deliberate.

Complex or restrictive rules are hard to stick to.

Diets filled with lists of good and bad foods are almost bound to get forgotten about over time.

Challenging exercise regimes with large amounts of time commitments and significant effort will become ignored when real life imposes its own priorities on you.

And complete abstinence from some of life's great pleasures is simply intolerable for most people, which is why the habits aren't designed to be followed seven days a week – just four.

And because the habits are so straightforward, I believe you will find them relatively simple to remember and ingrain into your life.

However, straightforward does not equate to easy. Making lifestyle changes can be extremely hard, which is why I am suggesting you phase in these changes over time.

But, taken together, and repeated consistently over time, I believe the five habits can have a profound effect on your life and health, and ultimately life expectancy.

Let's look at the five habits.

Habit 1: Have a breakfast that makes you feel fuller for longer

Foods rich in protein such as fish, meat or eggs will do this, as will whole grains (porridge being the prime example, although unsweetened muesli or Shredded Wheat® or bran also work). Feeling fuller for longer is important for when we get to habit 2, so you need to skip the pre-packaged cereals or a snatched round of toast as you dash out of the door. Cereals are full of processed carbs, as is bread, and your body will convert these into energy quickly, and you'll be hungry again by mid-morning.

Option one is therefore something like scrambled eggs with ham (or some smoked salmon if you are flush), or a boiled egg if you prefer. Or maybe full-on bacon and eggs. One egg doesn't feel enough for me, so I'd probably scramble a couple. Or prepare an omelette etc. Don't be tempted by bread/toast or hash browns though if you are going down this route as these processed carbs will spike your insulin levels (which we are trying to avoid doing).

However, I think a full cooked breakfast is a bit of a fussy, time-consuming way to start my day (certainly during the week), so for me the second option, the whole-grain route, is easier – so my habit is porridge.

One big scoop, with two scoops of skimmed milk. Three minutes in the microwave, a (small) dollop of jam, and I'm set. Jean, my wife, fluctuates between porridge and Weetabix®.

I also think that porridge or some form of bran is good for another reason. You are going to get protein every night on this plan, so ensuring you have some wholegrain everyday is also important as part of a balance in everything you consume.

Harvard School of Public health studied more than 100,000 Americans over 14 years, and found that a helping of whole grain every day (about 28 grams, the equivalent of

71

a small bowl of porridge) reduced mortality rates by 5%[xlv]. This was mainly due to a drop in cardio-vascular deaths of 9%.

Now this study probably found correlation rather than causation (i.e. if you are healthier, and therefore likely to live longer, you are probably already more likely to eat whole grains), but it was interesting nevertheless – and porridge it is for me.

Habit 2: Skip lunch

I'm going to explain later why taking extended breaks between meals can have such a beneficial effect – but it does.

Now you might be panicking here, thinking you can't go all day between meals. But you can. First, that's why you had a whole grain or egg based breakfast, in order to minimise spikes to your insulin levels, ensuring your body slowly releases energy from your breakfast during the morning and keep you full until and potentially beyond lunchtime.

And feeling a little hungry in the afternoon is no bad thing. You will feel the odd pang, but it soon passes, and actually over time those pangs do diminish.

If you really can't last until dinnertime, a handful of nuts are enough to keep you going later in the afternoon. I keep a bag in the car, in case I feel hungry on the way home, and a bagful in the kitchen for when I'm working from home. Just nuts though, not dried fruit (which is packed full of sugar, which isn't where we are heading). A handful is honestly all you need – and try to wait as long as you can before eating them (I might grab a handful around 4pm).

Again a recent very large scale Dutch study found that people who ate a handful or so of nuts every day lived longer[xlvi]. In fact, the drop in mortality was even stronger than the Harvard study on whole-grains. I suspect correlation again here too – but as with the whole grains, folk who live longer are clearly on to something, so grab some nuts.

Our ancestors probably skipped lunch most days for millions of years, so although psychologically daunting It really isn't that big a challenge when you actually have a crack at it.

And as I will explain later, this habit, like the others, is only Monday to Thursday – so lunch at the weekends is still OK!

Habit 3: Go for a walk

If you are comfortable with missing lunch, then instead of eating, go for a 30-minute brisk walk instead. It needs to be vigorous and purposeful though, rather than just a stroll. The evidence supporting walking as the "go to" exercise is becoming overwhelming[xlvii].

If walking at lunchtime is inconvenient, then aim to do 30 minutes at the start or end of the day. Again we are looking for four days a week, and ideally these will be the same days you are missing lunch, although frankly this is a habit you could do every day of the week.

Interestingly, brisk walking seems to operate just below the threshold at which your body cries out for a "post-exercise" feed. If you are a runner or cyclist/swimmer/gym-bunny, you will know that sensation, having finished a work-out, of feeling ravenous. That would be a problem here as I am asking you to avoid lunch. Walking though, does appear to sit below that level of intensity and so you shouldn't come back from your walk desperate for a snack.

Habit 4: For dinner, eat

- Good quality meat or fish
- Vegetables/salad
- Low or preferably no processed carbs

The good news is there's no "calorie counting" in this approach, and the very nature of the type of meals you should be preparing will mean you should always feel full at the end of the meal.

It's good, real food, and in portions big enough to keep you satisfied.

You can be much more flexible at the weekends – so those carbs you love aren't wholly off the agenda forever, But to be clear, by low-no carbs I'm principally talking about eliminating (or radically reducing) those dinner-time staples of white bread, pasta, white rice, potatoes (including chips), and other starchy carbohydrates from Monday to Thursday.

Outside of dinner of course this also includes eliminating sweets, snacks, crisps, biscuits and desserts. Also no sugar, fruit juice, dried fruits. And finally, stay clear of sliced, packaged meats.

I normally have an apple after dinner.

Habit 5: No booze, during the week (Monday to Thursday), at home

The Life of Riley habits are designed to let you lose weight if you need to, and get fit and physically active, and both goals are massively aided by not drinking every night.

Alcohol inhibits your body performing a chemical reaction known as lipolysis[xlviii] that is one of the key outcomes the plan is designed to trigger, so there is a perfectly logical health/diet/weight rationale for not drinking.

Some drinks also contain a lot of sugar (cider for example), which doesn't help if you are trying to cut down on sugar elsewhere, and they all contain some carbohydrates.

This habit therefore allows you (or orders you if you need a rule to stick to) not to drink for four nights a week under cover of "losing weight" or "getting fit", rather than because someone said you were hitting the bottle too much.

It might not sound clever if you aren't alcohol-dependent, but for someone like me, who was a heavy drinker, having the excuse that I'm not drinking for diet/fitness purposes allows me to leave the bottle unopened with fewer pangs.

Not drinking also stops you "overindulging" – i.e. not hitting the fridge late at night, slightly tipsy, searching for that secret stash of chocolate.

And those are the five habits.

I don't have a rule about coffee or tea. There's lots of research suggesting up to five cups of coffee per day is beneficial from a life-expectancy perspective, including a big study from the American Heart Association[xlix], although caffeine can stimulate insulin production which can get in the way of weight loss, so there's a balance here. Perhaps you might try to wean yourself onto one or two decaf cups a day.

I'd recommend you try to drink enough water not to be dehydrated – but as long as you are reasonably hydrated I don't think this is a critical issue, and good real food contains a lot of the water you need. Fizzy drinks and fruit juice should be treated with real caution too.

And that's it.

Five habits, phased in, followed by sensible application from there on.

1. wholegrain or egg-based breakfast;
2. no lunch;
3. go for a brisk walk instead;
4. good quality meat or fish with vegetables for dinner;
5. skip the alcohol.

And it's only Monday to Thursday.

The Weekend

"No pleasure is worth giving up for the sake of two more years in a geriatric home at Weston-super-Mare" Kingsley Amis

The great thing about *The Life of Riley* habits is we can avoid the curse of Kingsley – because, over time, you don't have to give up any pleasure (except smoking – which I'd argue is an addiction rather than a pleasure). At the weekends with *The Life of Riley* habits you can really relax – within reason – as your weight reduces.

You can eat out, have a drink, and enjoy a dessert every weekend, with the only proviso that you must be sensible. Don't overload on unhealthy processed food; don't binge drink to compensate for not drinking during the week; don't eat loads of snacks or desserts. If you can stick to the habits during the week, it should be reasonably clear how much extra flexibility you can allow yourself, whilst staying true to the overall goal of eating real food.

Chocolate is my weakness, and we continue to have some good quality stuff over the weekend as a treat, so there's no "hair shirt" going on here.

Timing

Phase 1 (months 1 to 3) – The warm-up

My good friend, the Psychologist Bill McAneny, said to me that there are two ways to change behaviours. The first way is to analyse the root causes of the bad behaviour, explain the impact of that bad behaviour to the person concerned, and outline the consequences of not changing, and then work together to build a plan to make changes over time so that behaviour eventually becomes modified.

The second way is just to tell someone to change his or her behaviour!

Being a CEO by trade, you'll not be surprised to hear me say I prefer route two.

As Bill said to me "...*This is all predicated on the fact that attitude does indeed determine behaviour, and that is usually where the focus tends to be, on changing attitudes that lead to behavioural change.*" However we often forget that behaviour also determines attitude. General George Patton was asked, in 1944 how he 'wins hearts and minds.' His answer is legendary and witty, but also incredibly profound. Patton said: "*Grab them by the balls and their hearts and minds will follow!..*"

Pushing the Patton imagery to one side just for a moment, that, in essence, is what I'm going to tell you about the five habits, given I can't analyse everyone individually. I'm just going to plough on assuming you'll come with me on this adventure. In the end, habits are simply behaviours that are repeated and so they become embedded and then instinctive. Think about a night out with your friends, it's 2.00am and you're really tired, you just want your bed, you need to sleep. But you don't do you? You brush your teeth! That is a habit, a behaviour that has been drummed into us since childhood, is repeated and so becomes instinctive.

There's a great metaphor you may have heard about how to overcome procrastination, which is borrowed from some Mark Twain quotes. In essence the advice is:

"If you have to eat a frog, do it first thing in the morning; and if you have to eat two frogs, eat the biggest/ugliest one first!"

So in real life this advice is to encourage you to tackle your biggest challenges head-first, and I think taken as a whole, changing five regular life habits counts as one of those big life challenges.

However, if you are going to try to change five habits, I'd suggest cracking them one or two at a time, and in a slight twist on the Mark Twain advice, getting the easier ones under your belt first to give you confidence before trying the tougher ones.

Some of those five habits will appear daunting to you. Maybe all of them do. The oft-quoted urban myth suggests we need to do something around 21 times before it becomes a regular habit. However, researchers at UCL discovered it takes longer, on average 66 days, before habits become automatic[1]. If we took all five habits in turn, and spent 66 days mastering each one individually, it would take almost a year to crack them all, which is clearly too long.

But if you are anything like me, when someone puts a new idea, thought or plan in front of you, and you like the look of it, you want to dive in straight-away, particularly if you want to hurry those results along. However, with *The Life of Riley* habits I think that would be a mistake, as there are just too many changes to cope with all at once in my view.

So, as a compromise, what I suggest is that over an initial three-month period, you gradually ease into the various habits of the plan, taking them one at a time. I was lucky when creating the plan that I had tried both a low carb eating regime before, and had also tried some fasting – so that meant I wasn't scared by combining those approaches.

I was also pretty good on the exercise front, so for me it was moving to porridge for breakfast rather than cereals or bread/toast/bagels (my former favourites), and quitting weeknight drinking that were the two new challenges. If you are faced with trying to implement multiple new lifestyle habits all at once, the whole thing might feel insurmountable, which is why phasing in the plan is such a critical idea.

So I'm going to suggest a particular order for warming-up into *The Life of Riley* habits, but feel free to juggle it around if you feel that would work better for you.

I'm going to assume here that having bought into the concept of the plan, you can immediately see the benefit from walking, and start to build that into your routine from the outset. You don't need to immediately do 4 days of 30 minutes from the get-go if you've never really walked in a structured way before – a gradual build-up to that level over the 3 months is fine.

But, in addition to developing your walking:

Month 1 – get stuck into the porridge/muesli/bran or eggs/ham/bacon etc. This isn't the most challenging change for most people I'd hope, but getting into a steady routine should give you a comfortable experience that making a change can become a permanent habit. And given I think it's a relatively easy change, hopefully having gotten half way or so to the 66 days on habit 1, you will have the confidence to move onto month 2.

Month 2 – stick with the breakfast changes and walking, but now add in skipping lunch. You might do this only once or twice for the first couple of weeks, moving on to three or four times as the month progresses – but as you'll already be consuming that healthier breakfast, you should find these days easier to cope with, and gradually they will become a habit. Even today, I don't normally manage four lunch-free days on the trot, simply because of work or social commitments, but I think I regularly manage three days off most weeks, and four once or twice a month. Don't beat yourself up if you can't do it everyday, but keep attempting it and you will eventually find yourself simply not thinking about lunch in the same "I must have some food" way. As this is month 2, I'm proposing here that you stick to your normal dinner plan, so you do have something you currently enjoy to look forward to in the evening, and are not fretting about getting dinner "right".

Month 3 – sticking with healthy breakfasts, walking and missing lunch, now go for the good quality meat or fish and vegetables dinner option. Cutting down on (or eliminating completely) carbs can be a shock to the system, but only initially.

As with month two, you might need to do this once or twice in weeks one and two, rising to three then four nights in weeks three and four. Even when carbs are still on the table, try to go for smaller portions. As this is still the warm-up phase, I am not here proposing you cut out the booze – get used to your new meal structure whilst enjoying a glass or two of wine or a beer if that's your regular routine.

Finally, after month three, move to stopping drinking during the week. Again you might want to only do two nights a week at first, although this habit change might be tough to do half-heartedly so I'd give the full four nights a go (for me this was the Mark Twain biggest frog challenge).

At this point not all of these habits will be automatic for you, but you will be well on the way with most of them.

You might want to change that initial order around to suit you, but I'm pretty confident that easing your way into the plan will mean by the end of the third or fourth month you are both raring to go, and not feeling nervous about your ability to stick with it going forward.

Habit	Month			Month
	1	2	3	4+
		The Warm Up		The Plan
Healthy breakfast	4-7	4-7	4-7	4-7
30 minute brisk walk	4-7	4-7	4-7	4-7
Skip lunch		2-3	3-4	4
Meat or fish + vegetable dinner			2-3	4
No booze				4

Numbers indicate frequency per week

The Plan (Month 4 onwards)

Once you are past the introductory phase, the number of days per week you need to stick to the habits is just four (but feel free to stick to the habits for five days per week if you want to motor along and aren't worried by stickbility).

The five Monday to Thursday habits are still sacrosanct, but you can ease back on Fridays, Saturdays and Sundays, so at the weekends:

- Stick to healthy breakfasts, but bacon and eggs or another cooked breakfast like this is probably more manageable on Saturday and/or Sunday for a touch of variety if you are following the whole grain option during the week.
- On Fridays, Saturdays and Sundays you can have both lunch and dinner if you want (I still don't eat lunch most Fridays – out of habit). You can let three of these six meals break the no-low carb habits, as long as you continue to eat real food and avoid processed foods such as pre-produced meals, fast food and snacks/sweets. Easing back on the bread, rice, pasta and potatoes is OK in moderation. There's a school of thought that only allows brown rice or wholemeal bread or wholemeal pasta for example when you are having a "carb" meal. Now I quite like wholemeal bread, but find brown rice and wholemeal pasta too fussy to cook, so I'd stick to white rice or plain pasta if I were having some.
- Sensibly, you should only have around four units of alcohol each evening, Friday to Sunday (that's two medium glasses of wine or two pints of beer) if you are using the habits to help you lose weight and drive your BMI down. I'm not going to get into age, sex or weight here. All will influence the amount that alcohol will affect you, but none of the evidence I have seen suggests four units a night, three nights a

week, is anything other than moderate. You should be your own judge.

- Enjoy an occasional treat such as a dessert or some chocolate, but again, don't go mad.
- Keep up the walking if you can at the weekends. If you do want to do something more exercise-intensive at the weekends, try to do it close to one of your "high-carb" meals, as your body will need to refuel at that time.

I'd stick with the plan in this form until your weight has reduced to the point where your BMI is 25 or under, based on the Trethefen graph highlighted earlier.

"High Performance – Low Maintenance"

When I was developing my ideas, and I showed the first iteration of *The Life of Riley* habits to anther diet expert, it simply said "do what you want" for the weekends. He was shocked, and probably quite rightly said I simply couldn't give people that much leeway when they were first starting out, as they could easily lose all the gains they had made if they weren't given some help to keep focussed during Friday, Saturday and Sunday. Hence the plan rules above.

But, once your BMI is 25 or below, you are now performing at a very high level, and really are into maintenance. And you will also be much more attuned as to how your body responds to changes in what you eat, or how much walking you do. This means you ought to be able to intuitively fine-tune the habits of the plan to build in a bit more weekend flexibility. So in this final, maintenance phase, there are no hard and fast guidelines for the weekends – which I think is a really key benefit of the plan, and one which substantially boosts its attractiveness.

But some things remain true. Monday to Thursdays should be sacrosanct – stick to those habits all the time. And if you want to continue to lose weight, or maintain your weight loss, eating desserts non-stop at the weekend will not help – so stick to one or two. Getting blotto every night will also challenge your power to not drink during the week, so don't tempt fate – but don't feel you can't occasionally have a drink or two, because you can. And once you are down to a BMI of 25 or below, you can enjoy a pizza or a burger on a Saturday night if you wish once in a while – or have an occasional carb-laden Sunday Roast for lunch if you want to. But you must balance the occasional blow-out by following it with a couple of really healthy days.

In general, taking a three day break from the Monday-Thursday regime is actually part of the plan – you actually need to loosen up a bit at the weekends so your body doesn't think you've ended up living permanently in a health farm. Just be sensible.

How regimented is the weekday element of the plan?

It's changing your lifestyle, so to that end, it's permanent – and that's pretty fixed. But can you flex within it if you need to? Of course you can.

Here are four things I occasionally do that break the habits.

1. Weeknight drinking. I only do this if I'm out with friends, or at a social event, and then normally only one glass. But please don't use this as an excuse to "socialise" every night of the week just in order to get some drink consumed! I might also have a drink on a Thursday or a Monday if it's a bank holiday weekend. But remember, I'm now down well below 25 on the BMI Scale, so I wouldn't relax this rule if you are still over 30 or just below.

2. Weeknight carbs. Of course vegetables contain carbohydrates, so this is not a no-carb plan, but one where the amount of carbs is radically reduced. Now I am at my ideal weight, I do enjoy some homemade chips

if I'm having a steak, or a spoonful of rice with a chicken curry or a stir-fry – but probably not every night. And I certainly try to get one or two meals per week done with none of the "big, bad carbs" at all (bread; pasta; rice; potatoes), preferably Monday and Tuesday. I certainly don't eat any meal that is primarily based around carbs though, such as pasta or pizza, during the week.

3. Weekday lunches – If you do have a job that requires the occasional lunch – try to schedule them for Fridays if you can. But, if you must go for lunch during the week, stick to fish and salad – no bread – no booze. No one will notice but you will not have broken the plan by much really on the odd day you do this.

4. Not going for a walk. If I'm working from home, time can quickly slip away, and I can get to the end of the day not having done anything. If that happens to you, just ensure that later in the week you can make up your missing 30 minutes.

Basically what I am saying here is these habits are meant for life – they should be the framework around which you live. But no-one can live that regimented an existence, so you are bound to break them from time to time. Just remember what they are, don't break them too often, and jump back on as soon as you can.

Holidays & Christmas

Let's be honest. Holidays & Christmas are a nightmare if you are trying to lose weight.

Well, the great thing about *The Life of Riley* habits is you can ease back for a week or two, and then hop straight back on. You'll discover your weight will go up a bit faster than it comes off – but so what – you're on holiday.

Including Christmas, I took about 8 weeks off in the first 12 months I was adopting these new habits and my weight went up an average of 1lb-2lbs per week during those periods "off plan" (although that did include a disastrous two weeks in North America, where we all know carbohydrate temptation lies in wait around every corner).

So weight probably goes on a bit more quickly than it comes off. Which makes sense given you are only really in full on "Habit" mode four days a week when you are on the plan, and you are probably not trying at all when you are off it on holiday.

Holidays are like extended weekends really, aren't they. So to that end, I would encourage you to take the sensible weekend approach when on holiday (i.e. don't have carbs with every meal), but run with that slightly looser regime for most of your break, and try to throw in one or two days each week where you fully stick to your new habits, avoiding lunch and going carb-free in the evening. I'd just encourage you to be sensible, and in particular to try to build in some exercise every day into your break. Holidays are great for walking, cycling, swimming etc. so really try to get a balance between letting your hair down and having a good time and keeping up some of your new habits.

And once you are back home living your habits the weight falls off again pretty quickly.

So *The Life of Riley* habits are flexible – but you do have to stick with it most of the time for it to work.

Can you vary it – skipping breakfast instead of lunch for example, or putting a "naughty" day in on Wednesday for example but being prudent on Friday? The answer is – I don't know, but I'd love to find out. Thelifeofrileybook.com website is designed to let you give me feedback on how you are managing with the habits – and if you want to try a variation – I'd love to hear about it. I'm currently trialling the plan with a number of volunteers, and will be reporting progress on the site from time to time, as well as blogging on the latest food, fitness, longevity and health issues, so please do check in to see the latest.

My advice for now though is to stick to the plan as

outlined above if you can.

In the end, if you want to cheat all the time, perhaps this plan isn't for you (but will any plan be?) I quite liked this quote from Peter Drucker *"...If you want something new, you have to stop doing something old..."*

There is a certain amount of self-discipline involved in any great endeavour – and you getting to the point where you are comfortably standing in Tribe 5 should be viewed that way, as a great endeavour. But before worrying about how you can cheat – give the plan a go in its entirety. You'll be surprised how straightforward it all is really.

In the next few chapters I'll explain what you need to do to fulfil all the habits, and how & why the plan works.

Chapter 7

"Food glorious food"

Lionel Bart (*Oliver!*)

I'm assuming here that during the week, you will eat dinner at home, so the habits are built around that perspective. For people who regularly eat out, you might need to think about how best to fit that lifestyle with this approach, but I think it can be done, as long as eating out means decent restaurants that serve meat, fish, vegetables and salads – and not fast food joints, which are disastrous for this type of eating regime.

Anyway, assuming you are doing the cooking, the meat and fish element of the habits just means a grilled (or pan-fried) chicken breast; or a salmon fillet; or a steak; or a pork chop; or a tuna fillet. All grilled or pan-fried – nothing too fancy – or even oven-baked for fish with vegetables for example – but feel free to add garlic, or chillies or other flavourings as required, although do be careful with highly calorific pre-packaged sauces etc. – steer clear of those. Olive oil works for pan-frying, as does butter, and I love sesame oil for its flavour in stir-frys.

I'm not doing a recipe book here – I assume you can find appropriate ways to select, cook and flavour foods without breaching the protein/ vegetable / low carbs-no carbs rule, but I have added a four week dinner schedule in Appendix 3 to give you an idea of how to approach your food planning.

In terms of general meat/fish quality, you must go for natural rather than processed such as pre-packaged burgers and sausages or fish fingers, although some traditionally preserved or cured meats are perfectly fine. You can make your own burgers at home and they are delicious. And try if you can to make oily fish a choice at least one night a week (tuna, salmon, trout, sardines) and another fish/seafood choice on another night as well (white fish, and/or prawns or other shellfish).

Of course you might not want to, or even be able to, spend the money on expensive cuts of meat for every night of the week. Less expensive cuts are fine too, and of course there are a variety of ways of cooking them that should allow you to stick to the guidelines above. Don't worry if these less expensive cuts are 'fattier". Fat in meat is fine. We've been eating it for millions of years.

Steamed or par-boiled for the veggies, or lightly fried in olive oil or butter if appropriate – fresh for the salad. Most sensible sauces for the salad (olive oil/balsamic vinegar is our default at home) are fine. I think legumes/beans in general are OK – you aren't likely to overdose on them – but be careful to avoid those that come in a can with a sauce. Ideally cook from raw if you can – but please be careful, as many legumes or beans or pulses need some soaking beforehand to be safe. Please read labels and check properly – I'm trying to keep you alive longer, not kill you.

Low carb is the key – and it means what it says. Ideally avoid dinner-plate carbs (pasta, rice, bread, potatoes, along with other processed carbs) altogether. You will get some carbs every day from dairy and vegetables, just not the very high proportion we now seem to be consuming in a typical western diet. However, I am a realist, and if you must have some, keep them to an absolute minimum. It can be a challenge if you are cooking for a family and there are other people you need to cater for who don't want to join the plan – so a modicum of will power might be needed to avoid eating their chips. If you are going to have some carbs, try to make them the smallest part of your plate. Remember too if you haven't had lunch you will feel hungry, so carbs on the table are tempting. So don't have them there at all if you can help it.

If you really want some extra carbs on top of dairy/vegetables – rather than rice try a little bit of a whole grain like quinoa (pronounced kinwa) – it has a nutty rice flavour, is high in protein, and is a pseudocereal, as it is actually related to spinach and beetroot rather than wheat. It tastes really good mixed in with a leafy salad, adding some more crunchiness to the vegetables. The other "trendy" option is cauliflower rice, where the cauliflower florets are whizzed in a food processor until they are as small as rice granules (or even a little smaller) and then gently pan-fried in butter for 6 to 7 minutes and used as a substitute for rice for curries, chillies and stir-frys.

The main message here though is good quality meat or fish and veg. And if it comes from a box, or is wrapped in cellophane – think twice about having it – most of the stuff you should be eating is produce you can buy loose from the supermarket, and most processed carbs come pre-packaged. Real food is the key.

I'd also be nervous about relying on pre-prepared meals, even those designed "to help you slim" – many of them are packed with bad trans-fats and sugars designed to add taste to food which has had the flavour removed by the processed cooking they've gone through.

Fresh is best – and I don't think this plan should test anyone's cooking skills – simple pan-frying or grilling, and some salad prep is not too challenging I'd hope.

But as I said, there's no emphasis on calorie counting, so eat until you are full. You are unlikely to massively over-indulge if most/all of your plate is good quality meat, fish and vegetables anyway.

I know current dietary advice is to moderate the amount of fat you consume. However, there's no real research to back this up as far as the healthy fats found in most meat and dairy products are concerned, so I'm pretty relaxed about it – as long as it's part of either the cut of meat or part of the cooking process or used as a dressing, or in some dairy element. I'd stick a chopped avocado into any salad once in a while to make it taste nicer, and cheesy cauliflower is always a winner for me. The old concern that high levels of fat lead to high cholesterol just hasn't been proven, and high cholesterol itself is not implicated in heart disease or shorter lifespans. As Science writer Matt Ridley summarised in an excellent *Times* leader recently *"... A 2013 review by the American Heart Association and the American College of Cardiology found 'no appreciable relationship between consumption of dietary cholesterol and serum [blood] cholesterol... Nor is there any good evidence that high blood cholesterol causes atherosclerosis, coronary heart disease or shorter life.'"*[li]

Now this relaxed approach to fat doesn't extend to trans-fats, which are a mainstay of much processed food. You might have guessed that no snacks are in the mix here. Sorry, but daily consumption of biscuits, cakes, sweets, crisps etc. is just not consistent with eating well. Anything with a high trans-fat or high sugar content is part of the problem, not the solution. End of story.

And do I need to say there are no puddings allowed during the week? Thought not. I do have a little bit of fruit in the evenings – normally an apple after dinner – but not too much. Most fruit is packed with sugar, so can defeat the low-carb approach, but one piece as a sweet end to a meal isn't going to kill you.

The sugary nature of fruit today is a worry I think. We're told to consume it in reasonably significant proportions, without any great scientific evidence. The "five a day message was dreamt up by someone without any scientific research to back it up, and is now a mainstay of our dietary thinking. Interestingly in other countries it is 7 a day, or even 10 a day, or a food pyramid – none with any worthwhile science to support them. For many people who are nevertheless trying to stick to five a day, fruit is probably easier than veggies to consume, especially as we are told fruit juice etc. counts (but in reality is really not great as it spikes your insulin). But I think you should forget five a day, and simply concentrate on eating a healthy amount of vegetables, and enjoy the occasional piece of fruit as a "dessert". It also appears too much fruit, spread throughout the day, can do lots of damage to your teeth[lii] as well as potentially undermining the low-carb approach outlined here.

And that overall food balance is pretty close to optimal I would say, and compares pretty favourably to the Mediterranean diet and other similarly lauded eating regimes.

I recently saw a great article called "simple habits for healthy eating" in the *NY Times* from Aaron E. Carroll, a professor of paediatrics at Indiana University School of Medicine[liii], which pretty much captured the whole Weekday Plan approach to food. Eating real food, as opposed to processed food, is the underlying key.

I'm grateful to obesity researcher Dr Zoë Harcombe for a great quote that captures much of this approach, and in particular how the manufacturers of processed foods have captured the health establishment and corrupted our approach to food. Her quote on food labels is *"I have a really simple food labelling policy – don't eat anything that needs a food label"*. Of course even natural foods like milk now come with labels so we are surrounded by the madness.

And the evidence for the greater effectiveness of eating real food, and in particular a regime which eliminates much of the processed carbohydrates in our western diet, in favour of a natural high-protein, high fibre, high-fat eating regime is quite compelling, as I will discuss in chapter 9.

I've posted a 4 week food plan in appendix 3 which gives you 16 different meals for 2 people. I'm no Jamie Oliver but most of the meals are pretty easy to cook and tasty.

92

Chapter 8

"You put the load right on me"

The Weight – The Band

One of the classic management rules is "if you can't measure it, you can't manage it". Thus was born the great management tool known as the "KPI" or Key Performance Indicator.

In laymans terms of course this just means having a target and measuring how close to it you are.

So for us, and the plan I am developing, over the next few chapters I'm going to set just three weekly targets for you to try to achieve, based on the habits. The first target is based on your Body Mass Index (BMI). This is essentially a measure of how much weight you are carrying, factored by your height, to give a roughly equal measure of "leanness/fatness" for everyone, irrespective of how short or tall they are.

The standard BMI measure is calculated by dividing your weight in kilograms by your height in metres squared. Unfortunately, although this is comparatively straightforward to work out, it's not the most accurate formula, especially for very tall people. Luckily a Cambridge mathematician, Nick Trethefen, came up with a slightly more complex formula, which produces much better results, so this does work better for bigger men in particular.

Rather than explain the formula to you, you can read about it online or check it out at thelifeofrileybook.com.

In addition, I've reproduced the simple graphic from chapter 2 in case you didn't check then and want to check now what your BMI is.

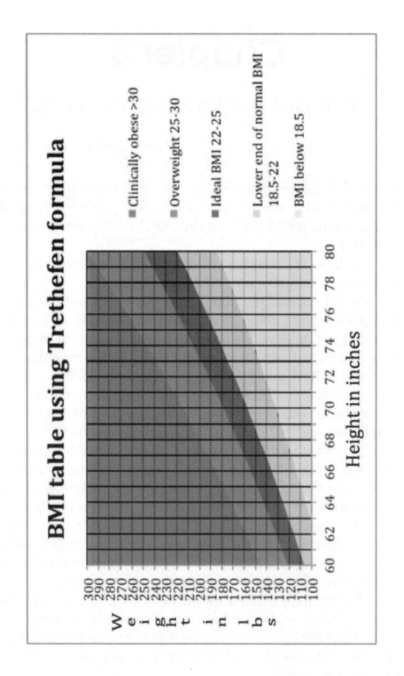

BMI table using Trethefen formula

Height in inches

Weight in lbs

- Clinically obese >30
- Overweight 25-30
- Ideal BMI 22-25
- Lower end of normal BMI 18.5-22
- BMI below 18.5

The BMI scale starts at 18.5 which is probably only of relevance for quite petite, lean women (some supermodels are around 17, which by common consent is frighteningly thin). Most men would struggle to get below 20, with even super-fit and skinny Tour de France cyclists only hitting this number at peak fitness. BMI scores can extend up to 40 and above for the heaviest amongst us. The key number here is 30, which is the benchmark for clinical obesity. You will either have a BMI greater than 30 or you won't. And if you do, the goal will be to get it down to 29.9 (or less, and I will list out a series of staged goals in a moment).

If your BMI is over 30, then you are clinically obese, and in the dark zone on the table. If that is the case, I would suggest checking out the online calculator on thelifeofrileybook.com website to get an accurate number. If it is over 35 then you are defined as being severely obese, and I'm afraid over 40 and you are morbidly obese.

Some business challenges are greater than others. I took a class at Columbia with a brilliant academic and entrepreneur, John O Whitney, who was a turnaround specialist. His job was to go into businesses on the verge of bankruptcy and save them – and he was very good at it too, and I'd like to think I learnt something from him. His primary rule in a turnaround was to do one thing – focus on the cash. If you had cash in the bank you were OK. If the cash ran out your goose was cooked.

This is the same for your weight. No matter what your BMI, that's your starting point – and if you are still here, reading this, you have some "'cash in the bank". John O Whitney's goal was to manage that cash, and use every (legal) trick in the book to increase the amount of cash the business had, thereby increasing it's survival chances. Your goal is the same. If your BMI is over 30, Every 1/10th of a point off your BMI is increasing your life expectancy, so driving that number down has to be your primary goal.

The target here is to get you to either a) drop down from the clinically obese BMI of 30+ if that's where you are starting and/or b) aim for a BMI in the mid 20s if you can, once you are below the 30 mark. I discuss BMI in some detail on thelifeofrileybook.com, and I do point out that there are flaws in the measurement. It is just one number, and it can be affected by lots of factors. But it's as good as we've got (and the Trethefen variation does help some of the odder results at the margins).

More importantly, it's the only continuous, large-scale data point researchers can look into at a population level to spot trends in weight-gain versus life-expectancy.

And to be clear, a BMI of 30.1 does not pose anywhere near the risk of a BMI of 40. In fact the data seems to suggest that compared to the population as a whole (many of whom are in that overweight category) each point above 30 is taking about a year off life expectancy, so it's only when you start to reach the mid-30s that it really begins to make a significant difference.

If you are currently clinically obese (or heavier), then by sticking to *The Life of Riley* habits I am confident you will eventually get to a weight you are comfortable with – and as long as your BMI is below 30 you will have moved out of Tribe 3 (and from "clinically obese" into the "overweight' category).

But – let's not stop there. I'd like to introduce you to the concept of the BHAG. I love BHAGs.

They are Big, Hairy Arsed Goals. The phrase was invented by a great business guru and author, Jim Collins, in his book *Built To Last* (if you're interested, you should also read his book *From Good To Great*)

They are the huge, life changing targets that can keep you motivated and challenged through the darkest hours of any project. Although he invented them for business, I think they apply to all of us, throughout our lives. We can all embrace BHAGs if we want to.

Perhaps the most famous BHAG was President Kennedy's speech to a joint session of the USA congress in 1961, where he said *"I believe that this nation should commit itself to achieving the goal, before this decade is out, of landing a man on the Moon and returning him safely to the Earth. No single space project in this period will be more impressive to mankind, or more important for the long-range exploration of space; and none will be so difficult or expensive to accomplish"*.

Wow.

I'm going to suggest you should adopt the same BHAG I gave myself at the start of developing *The Life of Riley* habits, when I discovered that the optimal BMI number for maximum life expectancy according to UK government data was 22.5. If you are very tall (like me), you must use the Trethefen formula rather than the standard one, because you could otherwise be giving yourself an unrealistic goal to aim at.

Your BHAG
To reach a BMI of 22-23

If you are over 60, you can stretch those numbers to 22 to 25.

If you already have that, or are so near as to make little difference, then move on, I'm talking to the rest of us now – those who can grab a little round the waist and hold on for a while.

And following on from that over-riding goal

Target 1 – to move your BMI
down each week

However, there's nothing worse than feeling you are

light years away from a target, and you can never get there. That's why psychologists (and good business leaders) will segment targets, and aim for incremental goals. So if your BMI is 33, whilst 23 can seem a lifetime away, I think we can place a number of milestones along the path to keep focussed, as the BMI data suggest certain neat dividing lines.

- Over 30 – clinical obesity – the first goal to crack is getting below this number
- 27.3 – the average UK BMI – getting below this would put you in the thinner half of the population. Double thumbs up for meeting this target
- 25 – the definition of "normal weight" is 25 and below – A great achievement when you get there.
- 22 to 23 – the optimal BMI for increased life expectancy, according to the data, for people under the age of 60. How fantastic will achieving this feel?

That's why it's target 1 and the BHAG of this book. The eating regime, drinking curtailment and physical activity in *The Life of Riley* habits are all designed to get you to this number as quickly and easily as possible.

Having had a BMI of 33, I have to say even after I first brought it down below 30, I ended up living for 15 years or so in the overweight category, with my BMI somewhere between 25-29 for most of that time. I was unhappy about being overweight without being miserable (and I suspect that's the same for most overweight people), but could never find the structure or diet approach that allowed me to get to the weight I felt I would be most comfortable at.

I do feel incredibly happy now however, with my weight down well below 15 stone and my BMI at 23, significantly below the "overweight" cut-off and almost perfectly in line with my own BHAG.

For me, feeling better at 23 might be because I enjoy cycling so much, and losing some weight does make climbing those hills a lot easier. Mind you, there are plenty of tubby cyclists out there, so not everyone appreciates speed going uphill, and it also goes to prove that it isn't exercise that makes you lose weight – it's eating the right foods in the right way.

And even ignoring life expectancy, losing weight over time is important. We hear a lot in the press about being "healthily obese" or, in tabloid terms "fat but fit". Sadly though, if you are healthy but obese now, the odds are it won't last. Research by the American College of Cardiology tracked 2,500 adults for 20 years tracking BMI, along with cholesterol, blood pressure and other indicators of health[liv]. The researchers defined the healthily obese as those with a BMI over 30, but with no other metabolic risk factors.

Over a 20-year period the research showed that more than half of the starting healthy obese participants became unhealthy. Only one in nine lost weight and became healthy, and the other 38% remained obese. That 50% shift to unhealthiness was far higher than what was observed in the healthy non-obese adults.

So if you have a BMI over 30, you need to get cracking to bring it down, and *The Life of Riley* habits contain all the ingredients to do just that.

Why did I specify "under 60" in the target for 22 to 23, and 22 to 25 for over 60s? Well, optimal BMI for life expectancy seems to rise a little as you get older, nudging towards 25 at age 60, and even over 25 as you get into older decades (70 and beyond). This is probably related to a bit of additional weight being useful in combating some chronic illnesses. If you are aiming to be in Tribe 5 however, you are hopefully a little less likely to succumb to chronic disease, so your optimal BMI ought to be 22 to 23 up to 60, and still be 25 or below even as you reach your 70s and 80s.

Chapter 9

"She blinded me with science"

She Blinded Me With Science - Thomas Dolby

If I were buying a "weight reduction" plan off the shelves of my local supermarket, I'd want to know the answers to three questions.

1. Is it scientifically sensible and safe (validity)?
2. Is it maintainable over a long period (sustainability)?
3. Does it actually work (efficacy)?

So, how well should *The Life of Riley* habits work in helping you to lose weight, and why do they work at all?

If you were to give the plan a pseudo-scientific title, it would probably be called

"a composite neo-low carbohydrate-intermittent fasting regime, with scheduled furloughs combined with regular moderate metabolism-raising physical activity".

I think *The Life of Riley* habits works better as a name.

And before we get into the details, I do need to tell you it's working brilliantly for me.

Of course if you are currently suffering from any medical condition, you should always consult your doctor before embarking on a new regime.

Validity

The science of weight gain and weight loss is imperfectly understood. You could surf the internet for hours and find masses of conflicting views and opinions. Body chemistry is complex, so the interaction of blood sugars, insulin, fats, gut bacteria etc. is challenging to understand.

Some scientists are starting to research genetic differences within populations, to see whether some people would be better on one type of diet, and other folk on a different one. That would be a major breakthrough if it turned out to be accurate. Other scientists are investigating gut bacteria, and think some people are missing some healthy bacteria that, if added back, could halt and potentially reverse obesity. Again – fantastic if it turns out to be scientifically possible – but something for the future, rather than the present.

I am not a scientist. But I think I am capable of reading the scientific literature and coming to some sensible conclusions. However, like you, I probably started off being bewildered by it all. The sheer number of different diet approaches (low-cal, low-carb, paleo, high fat, low fat, ketogenic etc.) can be bewildering. Some meta-analysis[lv] suggests that they "all work" to some degree, but that the difference is found in the "stickability" or ability to adhere to the regimes.

However, more recent evidence suggests that not all diet approaches are created equally. In fact, given the number of us permanently on a diet, and the sheer number of overweight and obese living among us, I'd be tempted to say most approaches don't work to any appreciable degree at all.

Let's be clear. Obesity has rocketed in the past 40 years, from an inconsequentially low number to over a quarter of the population, despite us being obsessed by diets, getting fit etc. And those odds on being able to come back down from obesity (over 1 in 200 for men, 1 in 125 for women) are frightening (if true), so something serious has been going wrong, and the received wisdom on how to tackle it by dieting doesn't seem to be working.

There are two main types of weight loss programmes – low-fat and low-carb – and the evidence is now pretty conclusive that low-carb is the way to go for most people. A major report in 2015, published in *The Lancet*, and widely reported, including here in *The Guardian*[lvi] was clear that low-fat diets did not work well, and that low-carb had a statistically better effect. *"There is no good evidence for recommending low-fat diets,"* said lead author Dr Deirdre Tobias from Brigham and Women's Hospital and Harvard medical school, Boston.

However, the problem for low-carb diets (along with all weight-loss programmes) is "stickability", with most people giving up well before a year on any plan, limiting effectiveness.

We'll come back to "stickability" in a moment – but first, why does low-carb work, and is there anything that can boost its effectiveness.

Low-Carb

The rise in obesity has occurred at around the same time as two related changes in our food consumption patterns. First, western governments changed their dietary advice to recommend eating less fat and more carbohydrates, and second, the giant food manufacturers seem to have gained a stranglehold on our food consumption, both in and out of home. The data doesn't suggest we are eating more food than we used to – just that more of it is carbohydrate based, and in particular, more of it comes in the form of pre-packaged, processed carbs. From all of the evidence I have seen it is the increasingly regular consumption of carbohydrates, and in particular processed carbohydrates that is making us fat.

When constantly replenished by regular carbohydrate intake (sandwiches for lunch, snacks and biscuits during the day, pasta or rice or chips for dinner etc.) your body will rarely run out of its easiest energy source. So you are keeping your engine fully topped up and raring to go. Scientist Valter Longo, who works for Southern California's longevity institute, likens this approach to *"...driving along with your foot constantly hard on the accelerator pedal."*

Carbs are easy for the body to break down into glucose. Consuming carbs (or sugar) also triggers the release of insulin. Your body converts the carbs (or sugar) into glucose, which insulin then helps convert into usable energy. However, the glucose not used for energy is also easy to lay down as fat. If athletes "carb-load' before a long bike ride or big run – why do the rest of us also "carb-load" before a night sitting in front of the TV? All we are doing is helping to lay down fat.

However, if you avoid or significantly reduce carbohydrates over an extended period, this dramatically lowers your insulin levels. Insulin is the chemical that helps muscles use those carbohydrates (and sugars) you consume as energy within the body. It also inhibits the body using fat stores as an energy source. Over time, avoiding carbohydrates reduces glucose in your body, in turn reducing insulin. This lack of glucose in your body (and therefore lack of insulin) triggers a mechanism known as lipolysis, which essentially forces your body to dip into its fat reserves to keep your energy levels up, producing chemicals known as ketones as a by product (unfortunately these can give you slightly bad breath, so an investment in sugar-free mints or gum may be required here!)

So, if you want to reduce fat, this is the only way you can do it. Just cutting back on food intake willy-nilly simply isn't guaranteed to trigger the chemical processes required to shift your body into using its body-fat reserves.

Now any calorie-controlled diet is likely to lead to some reduction in the amount of carbs you consume, helping to potentially create the conditions for short-term fat loss. But just reducing calories doesn't specifically target that fat-loss mechanism, and therefore a simple low-fat or calorie counting approach is doomed to failure from the start. Your body adjusts to you reducing your energy intake by reducing the amount of energy it needs (cutting back on essential maintenance for one thing) and you haven't fully triggered any fat-loss mechanism, so the calorie deficit never converts to much reduced weight. And it also causes you to obsess over food, because you are starving. So once you slip off that calorie controlled diet, wham, back you are over-eating the wrong foods and putting the weight back on.

The whole "reduce your calories and you will lose weight" formula just doesn't work either. Protein requires much more effort by your body to digest and consume than carbohydrates or fat do. So any fixed calorie controlled diet can mean you end up with widely varying amounts of "usable" calories depending upon the mix of food you are consuming. And given the calorie deficits people on these diets are supposed to be achieving, they should be losing far, far more weight than they do. If you could cut back by 500 calories a day every day for a year, according to the "less energy in vs. same/more energy out = weight loss" theory you should be reducing your intake by 3,500 calories per week, which is approximately 1lb of energy. So at the end of the year if you keep up normal energy out levels, you'll have lost 52 lbs – or almost 4 stone. Yet do you know many people who have achieved this level of weight loss through calorie control alone? Thought not. The reason those "slimmers of the year" make the front page of the papers is because they are so rare. One person might lose a significant amount of weight this way – but millions don't. Nutritionist and food researcher Dr Zoë Harcombe has written extensively about this on her blog if you want more information[lvii].

Hence the rave reviews for diets such as Atkins and South Beach when they first emerged, which overturned conventional thinking as they didn't calorie count, and instead specifically blocked carbohydrate intake and forced your body into lipolysis or even ketosis (which is a very specific biological state). Most low-carb diets are known as "ketogenic" for this reason.

In addition to that meta-study I referred to at the start of this chapter, there are any number of studies that show that low-carb diets work better than low calorie diets in terms of weight loss and almost universally resulted in better measures for other key health indicators such as blood pressure.

One 2001 study at Duke University[lviii] came to the simple but profound conclusion "Compared with a low-fat diet, a low-carbohydrate diet program had better participant retention and greater weight loss".

The numbers were quite compelling – 26lbs lost on average for the low-carb group vs. 14lbs for the low-fat group, with 76% of the low-carb participants sticking with the plan for the full 24 weeks vs. only 57% of the low-fat dieters. Both groups lost around the same proportion of fat (74%-78% of the total loss).

Interestingly the high-protein/low-carb group weren't told to reduce the total amount of food (measured in calories) they were to eat, but they ended up eating an almost identical number of calories anyway compared to the low-fat group who were told to restrict their diet. I do think your body naturally controls the amount you consume on a low-carb diet, meaning you don't over-eat. Carbs are very "more-ish" aren't they? And given the higher effort required to digest the greater amount of protein, you are inevitably running "more efficiently" despite not feeling hungry on a high-protein/low-carb diet.

The change in bodily chemistry was demonstrated in the Duke research by testing urine samples from the low-carb group. The number showing some ketones in their urine was markedly higher after just two weeks on the regime (86%). Higher levels of ketones in the urine indicate that the body is using fat rather than carbohydrates or sugar as its primary source of energy.

Admittedly this was just one study, but plenty of others suggest low-carb has the edge in terms of both the size of weight loss, and more importantly the ability to stick to the plan. One weblink[lix] provides a useful summary of over 23 randomised controlled trials, all published in respected, peer-reviewed journals, showing measurable, statistically significant benefits of low-carb over low-fat diets.

Can the low-carb approach be boosted? I think it can.

Intermittent Fasting

This is a new approach to eating which is gathering adherents, and seems to have a measure of scientific logic and evidence to support it.

As well as reduced carbohydrate intake triggering lipolysis, it can also be encouraged by fasting, which obviously ends up with your body emptying itself of carbohydrates, as you are going longer periods between food intake.

The Life of Riley habit of skipping lunch isn't full-blown fasting of the type suggested by some converts to massive calorie restriction, but building in a good 11-12 hour buffer each day between meals seems to have a positive effect on our bodies, and not just in terms of weight-loss.

In a test on mice there was a dramatic difference in the outcomes when the mice were split into two groups, fed the same diet, but with one group restricted in their feeding to just one eight-hour window per day[lx]. The difference in the results was amazing, and to quote from the paper's summary *"Mice under time restricted feeding… are protected against obesity, hyperinsulinemia, hepatic steatosis, and inflammation and have improved motor coordination ... These changes in catabolic and anabolic pathways ... improved nutrient utilization and energy expenditure."*

OK – a bit scientific – but quite a long list of health benefits for the mice concerned, and perhaps suggestive that fasting for a while every day might provide you with something beneficial too. This of course is the complete opposite of the "eat something little and often" approach.

Scientist Valter Longo thinks intermittent fasting appears to switch on a number of DNA repair genes, shifting the body from growth mode to repair mode.

If lipolysis is triggered by reducing carbohydrate intake, and is enhanced by fasting, you are giving yourself probably up to four days a week of fat reduction on *The Life of Riley* habits.

Other scientists have looked at intermittent fasting vs. low-calorie dieting and come to similar conclusions about its efficacy. However their approach mandates quite low calorie intake during fasting days (some suggest alternate days only consuming 500-600 calories, others a 5:2 approach, with 2 fasting days per week at the same level), whereas *The Life of Riley* habits simply build in a series of long, 12 hour fasting periods within a reduced carbohydrate intake over a four day continuous period.

I'm not sure you need to combine extended non-eating windows with low-carb meals and then make those meals tiny – that seems to me to be a triple-whammy that would be mighty difficult to maintain. I think getting into "fat being used for energy" mode each week is more important, hence my recommendation not to count calories for your evening meal, but rather let the style of meal (low carb) naturally and healthily moderate your food intake.

Some people who have bought into this "time restricted" plan only eat lunch and dinner, thereby keeping their food intake to a restricted 8-hour window (like the mice I guess). Good if it works. But I'm not sure I'm convinced you need to do that – I don't think it fits with the evolutionary principles I will outline in a moment, and I think it would be really hard for most people to maintain, as breakfast and dinner are probably the two most ingrained meals of the day. Also, I'm walking at lunchtime, so lunch is off the menu for me! But if you fancy lunch instead of breakfast, give it a go if you can stick to healthy low carb eating. I know some people who only eat one meal per day. That is a display of amazing self-control.

So if low-carb and intermittent fasting are both having the same effect, combining them ought to provide a powerful positive feedback loop. But is there any reason why we should combine them?

I'm a big fan of going back to evolutionary principles in thinking about these matters, and it seems to me perfectly logical that our ancestors, for millions of years a) didn't consume processed carbs because they simply weren't available, and b) went for long periods each day unable to eat much as they were out hunting and gathering, and that a two meals a day strategy, morning and evening, fits that pattern. Even more recently, I suspect lunch was something reserved for the richest in society, and that most of our ancestors right up until just a few years ago focussed on breakfast and evening meal only, with a diet rich in protein, fat and vegetables/fibre.

Interestingly fruit doesn't feature too highly in my focus here (despite the government's "five a day" mantra). And I think there's a rather counter-intuitive evolutionary reason why fruit should be treated with a little caution. Even though one could imagine our ancestors eating fruit, this would only have been in season, and wild, uncultivated fruit was likely to have been much, much lower in sugar (which remember triggers insulin production) and higher in fibre than the fruits commercially grown today. I'm also not a fan of "juicing" as it seems to me this simply rips most of the fibre out of the fruit and vegetables, which is half the reason for eating them.

So the science supports these two approaches, neither of which seem to me to be at all risky from a health perspective (unlike many diet regimes out there involving pills, powders and potions for example, or non-stop juicing, or dropping large amounts of butter into coffee for breakfast), and combining them seems to me to be pretty logical.

And the beauty of *The Life of Riley* habits is you are only being really "careful" for four days at a time, so even if you are reducing your total food intake compared to your previous norms, your body doesn't have time to register the reduction and reduce your metabolism to respond (especially if you are busy walking everyday). The massive reduction in processed carbs from Monday-Thursday does the trick of triggering the use of fats to fuel your body, and having some carbs on Friday to Sunday allows you a safety valve.

The Life of Riley habits have two elements that naturally limit the opportunities for you to make bad food choices. First you aren't eating lunch, and lunch for most people at work tends to be shop bought, and highly carb based (sandwiches, pasta salads etc.), and secondly a high protein/fibre/fat evening meal will leave you feeling full without any need to over-indulge. So there's no real need to calorie count, and you don't need to worry about the steak being too big. And of course cutting out the booze also massively reduces your "empty calorie" intake.

That's the simple explanation of the plan. And everyone will react differently. But it seems to work.

Sustainability

Onto my second question. Although the science behind "low carb" dieting, augmented by some low-impact fasting works, what about the second of my questions – how easy will it be to stick to

We all know that diets that restrict your overall food intake are hard to stick to, for powerful biological reasons[lxi], particularly for those who are over-eating for complex emotional reasons, hence the need for communal support via voluntary groups or commercial diet organisations. I'm not knocking these communal weight-loss approaches – for some people they will be perfect if they promote the consumption of the right foods, although I'm not convinced any approach that still has you eating a lot of carbs as a percentage of your food intake, or limiting the amount of food you eat is going to work effectively.

For others though, like me (and perhaps most men), we've just ended up too heavy, and want to shift the weight off as quickly and efficiently as possible, and whatever approach we take, it's got to be something we can live with long enough for it to work.

Those generic "low carb" diets were a highly successful innovation in weight-loss when they first emerged – because they worked, and promised freedom from small helpings and counting. Atkins took the west by storm, and was followed by Scarsdale etc.

But I think they are all just too hard to stick to for any sustained length of time (perhaps they become just dull and boring?) Many friends of mine had good early success, then fell off the wagon. They were too repetitive for me, which is why although they worked for me in losing weight to begin with, I gave up quite quickly and ended up regaining some of my initial losses, just as that meta-study predicted. Being denied carbs completely seems to me to be a sacrifice too far. The occasional rice or pasta dish seems to be one of life's great pleasures, especially if one uses good quality ingredients, and even sneaking the odd bag of crisps or biscuit from time to time (at the weekend) isn't going to kill you.

Then fasting diets took over – again because they worked (for similar reasons to low carb as they both trigger similar bodily responses) and because for four or five days a week, you were free to eat what you wanted. Again though, fasting for an entire day, with very low calorie intake for evening meals, two or three times a week is challenging. The fasting diet worked for me again for a while, but I found the fasting days just a bit too tough, perhaps because at the time I weighed 16-17 stone, so living on 500-600 calories was just too brutal for my body to bear. I was also uncomfortable that on the other days I was effectively being given licence to eat "junk" if I wanted – that just seemed wrong.

The beauty of *The Life of Riley* habits is they avoid both of these traps. There isn't a "calorie count" attached to them; you are not locked into the slightly restrictive element seven days a week; and you are encouraged to eat good, real food all of the time.

So *The Life of Riley* habits sample the best from both the low-carb and the fasting approaches, and not only combine it with a surreptitious alcohol-reduction programme, but also throws in a fitness boost to boot.

So there's no calorie counting, and you get to eat a full meal every night, and you get essentially three days a week with more flexibility within the regime anyway. And you can skip a day here and there if you need to. And you can have Christmas and holidays off too. I can't think of any other eating regime/diet plan which has that amount of "stickability" built in. Of course there are downsides (restricted breakfast options, no lunch or booze four days a week, low carbs four days a week) but compared to the relentlessness of some of the mainstream diets, *The Life of Riley* habits have a lot going for them.

I clearly haven't done any large scale trials, so I'm an experiment of one (well, two actually including Mrs R) – but I'm not feeling any pressure to break the plan, and haven't since the moment I started it well over a year ago. I'm not on it for three days a week anyway, and I know I will come off for holidays, Christmas etc. And I can come off for a day or so in the week whenever I want if there's a special occasion, because I know I will be back on the next day.

As long as you know this is going to be your "routine" then there's no real pressure about it. I think that is the key – this isn't a diet, it's a new way of life, so it has to be able to work long-term, and it has to be able to cope with the vagaries of living in the modern world.

I've rarely felt hungry, except occasionally during the middle of the afternoon, but I've known I was going home to a steak, or a nice roast chicken, so that feeling soon passes – or I grab a handful of nuts and I'm sorted.

It's also true that constant yoyo dieting, and shifting large amounts of weight on and off can place strain on your body – so whatever you do needs to be sensible, and maintainable. Which I think is why *The Life of Riley* habits are so good, because the weight does come off regularly and smoothly, and the plan itself is maintainable.

The one point I would make here (as well of course as checking with your doctor if you have a health condition) is not to try to combine this with any really intensive sports-training, as you will be putting yourself into a severe calorie deficit at that point. Walking seems to be fine, as it doesn't trigger any huge bodily demand for energy intake, but if you are training for a marathon, or are a regular gym bunny, you will need to alter the amount and timing of your food intake accordingly, so you can refuel properly close to the end of exercise.

Any serious fitness activity probably also means you will be tempted to use carbs as part of your refuelling. Although refuelling on fat is far more effective, I find a craving for carbs (a buttered bagel for example) just after a long bike ride is hard to resist. If you do consume increased amounts of carbs, this is likely to alter the timing and intensity of any lipolysis effects. For this reason I do try to keep my more intensive activity (my once a week gym session, or cycling for example) to the weekend where a bit of carb-based refuelling isn't interfering with the basic structure of *The Life of Riley* habits.

Efficacy

So on to my final question. Does it work?

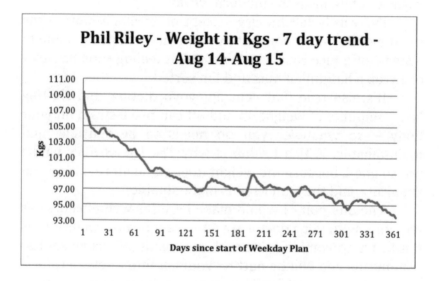

Here's the report after one year on the plan.

I am writing this chapter on Monday 2nd August 2015. I initiated the plan on Tuesday 26th August 2014. So I've been running with this for a total of 49 weeks, but a net of 41 weeks, due to breaks, holidays etc.. I stopped completely for two weeks over Christmas, and for two weeks during a holiday in February (that big upwards spike around day 180 is the effect of 10 days in the USA & Canada) and two weeks during a break in April.

I have lost 37 lbs. during the active 41 weeks. So just under 1lb per week.

My BMI (which at one stage in my life was over 33) has dropped from 27 to under 23 in 11 months, moving me out of "overweight", through "normal" weight, to the ideal number.

My body fat % has dropped from 26% to 20% – again well into "normal" territory.

Remember, I am 6ft 5ins tall, and used to weigh over 20 stone at my peak. My weight is now a new low of 14st 8lbs. Truly a momentous day.

Up until last month, I had not seen the number 14 at the left of my scales for at least 20 years – if not longer. When I was at my heaviest, in 2000, I was over 20 stone, and I imagine it took me at least 5 years or more to put that amount of weight on, so I can't have been below 15st since the mid-nineties at the latest. I can't recall my youthful weight but I was pretty thin in my teens and 20s, so I think I can recall a 13st period – but I'm not sure – and that would have been in the 1970s/80s anyway.

But 14st something is brilliant. And my goal is to keep it under 15st from now on.

You should never of course reveal a lady's age, or weight, so all I will confirm about my fellow-traveller in this, my wife Jean, is that she now also has the magic BMI number of 22.5 – which she is quite chuffed about too.

So yes – it does work – at least for us, and I would be amazed if this approach didn't work for the vast majority of people who tried it.

Chapter 10

"There's people livin' in the bottle"

The Bottle – Gil Scott-Heron

Here's another quote from my favourite business guru, Peter Drucker *"Unless commitment is made, there are only promises and hopes... but no plans."*

For me, reducing the scale of my own drinking has been the hardest part of the plan. I was, without doubt, a heavy/frequent drinker. I drank a bottle of wine most, if not every, night of the week. And I was doing it for so long I can't ever remember a time when I didn't drink that much most nights. Now I have weighed between 15st and 20st for most of my adult life – so I can absorb a lot of alcohol – there's a lot of blood to dilute it! And I only ever ended up feeling tipsy after a bottle. I was always fresh the following morning – no hangovers from a decent Rioja they claim, and the predominant personality change was to make me even more annoyingly argumentative round the dinner table. So I was fine, I told myself.

And I regularly did "dry January" proving to myself that I wasn't addicted because I could go an entire month without the booze. And I could (although I used to shorten it to 28 days so I could get back to the drink!)

But I was drinking a bottle a night. And my kids were nagging me; and I wanted to lose the weight; and then I started doing the research for this book – and then I knew I simply had to find a hook to hang not drinking on.

So *The Life of Riley* habits work for me. I don't drink because I'm in weight loss/weight maintenance mode

Monday to Thursday, and the alcohol would play havoc with that. But really, I know I just need to stop consuming it every night for the sake of my liver. And I feel a lot, lot better for it.

Don't get me wrong – I still want a glass most nights – I just know I couldn't stop at just one, so I have none. Unless I'm out, when I will have a glass, but then only one because I'm probably driving, or with guests/clients etc. so need to remain sober.

And that is the beauty of a plan or set of habits which you know are a permanent, good feature of your life – you can skip them once in a while and not feel concerned, because you know the plan is still there for you when you restart it the following day.

If you are genuinely addicted, you will not be able to survive more than a day or two without the booze before having severe withdrawal symptoms. If that is the case you should seek professional help.

However, if you can go for one, two, three and then four days without feeling physically ill, you are probably like me, and a large number of other people in being more psychologically than physically dependent, and using it as a lifestyle habit, and probably ignoring the harsh side-effects. You need to break the daily habit/routine – you need some form of rule which simply stops you opening the bottle. *The Life of Riley* habit of not drinking during the weekday evenings allows you to do that.

If you are a "social" boozer, i.e. you head down the pub every night for a quick one before heading home, I'm afraid you are going to have to alter your routine. You don't need to envisage a life without the noise, warmth and camaraderie of your local; you just need to walk on by during the week.

So better to have some structure which can easily take care of that. And I know of many people who already simply don't drink "on a school night", and have actually adopted habit 5 of the plan as a staple of their lives.

Only you can make the mental break in order to slow

down your drinking, but it really is worth it.

The stats for life expectancy for alcohol dependent people, especially the high number of older men, are frightening really.

The temporary abstinence I am proposing within *The Life of Riley* habits approach is a fast-growing trend on both sides of the Atlantic. In the USA, many folk who recognise they have an alcohol dependency problem have moved to a similar structure to *The Life of Riley* habits, known as Moderation Management (MM). This approach was the subject of a recent *The Guardian* online article[lxii]. Not without its critics, it does however seem to me to be a very useful way to address heavy drinking without forcing people into full abstinence in a way they find impossible to maintain. One of the MM directors, Marc Kern, has written a book on the topic of responsible drinking if you want to know more.

Here in the UK organisations like Soberistas and Hello Sunday Morning are doing similar work.

And the abstinence built into *The Life of Riley* habits is not a life sentence. Unlike smoking, which I do believe you have to stop completely, drinking two or three nights a week seems to be a far, far smaller risk to your health than true dependency, if not actually positive from a longevity perspective. You are effectively giving your liver a rest from when you wake up Monday morning through until Friday night, every week. And like your lungs, health scientists think the liver has great powers of recuperation, as long as it's not irreversibly damaged.

And here's the good news. As well as not drinking Monday to Thursday being great for your liver, drinking on the weekend in sensible amounts seems to be good for your life expectancy.

Moderate Drinking

Moderate drinking has been linked in many studies with positive health benefits, and this fact was noticed over 20 years ago by the doyen of epidemiology (the study of big medical data sets), Sir Richard Doll[lxiii].

Author and Director of Lifestyle Economics at the IEA Christopher Snowden is leading the charge in favour of moderate drinking[lxiv], and many studies do seem to show that moderate drinkers have better life expectancy than "never-drinkers" (i.e. by comparing them to people who have never drunk at all, and excluding those who were drinkers but have given up, who may be in poor health already). And remembering what I said earlier about people misusing statistics, watch out for spurious articles dissecting the data to prove alcohol doesn't have health benefits[lxv].

One study in particular showed that healthy men (i.e. those who didn't smoke, exercised regularly and were not obese) who drank moderately had a much lower risk of coronary heart disease than those who had never drunk[lxvi]. This does fit perfectly into the structure of *The Life of Riley* habits. Other studies[lxvii] show similar effects.

One major meta-study, published in the *Journal of the American Medical Association* (*JAMA*), showed the effect of moderate drinking vs. total abstinence and binge drinking. This was a pretty big study of over 1m people across America, Europe and elsewhere[lxviii].

The lowest mortality rates were associated with half to one "drink" per day, but reduced mortality compared to non-drinkers was still visible at up to four "drinks" per day. The scientists themselves, who split the data between men and women, suggested the optimal results in terms of reduced mortality were for up to two "drinks" per day for women, and three "drinks" per day for men. In this study, a "drink" equals 10 grams of ethanol, which is slightly higher than the UK unit measure (which is 8 grams of ethanol). Converting those "US daily drinks" into weekly UK units would suggest up to 18 units for women and 26 units for men per week was associated with reduced mortality compared to complete abstinence. These levels are a touch higher than the old (2015) UK suggested limits of 14 units for women and 21 for men, but are not noticeably different in totality.

The study provides a very useful conclusion – to quote "...this meta-analysis confirms the hazards of excess drinking but also indicates the existence of potential windows of alcohol intake that may confer a net beneficial effect of drinking, at least in terms of survival, both in men and in women. Heavy drinkers should be urged to cut their consumption, but people who already regularly consume low to moderate amounts of alcohol should be encouraged to continue."

All of the studies here were "self reported" – i.e. the researchers were basing their results on what people told them they had drunk. As we know from the Liverpool John Moores University study I quoted earlier and this USA research[lxix], people routinely under-report their drinking levels when asked, probably by between one third and a half. In practice this almost certainly means that the actual levels of "safe' drinking, i.e. drinking associated with lower levels of mortality, is potentially higher than two "drinks" per day for a woman, and three "drinks" per day for a man – so we've got some wiggle room, even on these levels, as this blog post from Christopher Snowden, highlighting a letter to *The Guardian* from Robert East, Professor emeritus at Kingston University, confirms[lxx].

So if we want to be moderate drinkers, what does that mean on a practical basis for how much we should consume? Well we start with a huge problem in that I doubt anyone in the general pubic can accurately define what a unit of alcohol is, and as we can already see from the UKs 8 grams of ethanol per unit vs. the USA meta-analysis being based on 10 grams per "drink", it is a pretty arbitrary amount. Let's assume, for the sake of argument, the widely agreed base that a normal 750 cl bottle of wine is 10 UK units (some stronger, full bodied reds might be more, some dry whites less, which is another complication which we will skip for now). This is a pretty accurate number according to most alcohol researchers. So 75 cl is 1 unit. But no one drinks wine in 75 cl measures. A medium glass in a pub is supposed to be 175cl – so that's 2.3 units. A large glass is 250 cl – so that's 3.3 units. So that's not helpful. You're not going to keep 2.3 or 3.3 readily in your mind next time you nip down to the pub – and when you are at home, filling up your glass, do you have any idea what the measure is?

And once we've established how much we are drinking – what should the right limits be? You might be worried about just reading lines off a graph, and therefore think government recommendations might be a better guide. Well, the old (up to 2015) UK government advice for women was two to three units a night, with 14 units per week overall. Now I don't want to be picky but three units is 50% more than two – a pretty wide margin. For men the old advice was up to three to four units per night (with 21 units overall), a 33% gap.

Let's be brave and assume three units is alright for a woman in one session. So a single large glass is technically too much, and two medium glasses is way over.

For a man three to four units was the recommended amount per drinking session. Let's go large and assume four units was OK. So for him a single large glass wasn't quite at his limit, but two medium glasses was again a little too much.

And the same pedantic calculations can be made for beer and spirits.

Flipping heck, as my mum would have said, what a palaver. This whole business is hard enough without having to remember drinks with decimal places, and boundaries and gaps, and adding back what you drank a couple of nights ago. People need simple advice, and for it to be made relevant to what we consume.

The whole units thing is a bit of a disaster really, particularly from a marketing perspective if you were a public health official tasked with communicating this to the public. It is especially bad because there's not an easy read across from wine to beer to spirits. A pint of beer is worse than a single large glass of wine, but not as bad as two medium glasses. By now we're all saying "give me a break", or should that be "give me a drink".

And this is before we've considered that some beers are more alcoholic than others, as are some wines. And the fact that people of different sizes clearly have a different capacity to safely absorb the booze in the first place. I weigh 94 Kg, but could weigh 100Kg and still be considered normal weight. A small woman of around 5ft 5ins could weigh as little as 50 Kg and also be of normal weight. But I am literally twice her mass. One size clearly doesn't fit all as far as booze recommendations go.

The "unit" based approach to how much you can consume each week was of course just "an intelligent guess" (or picked out of thin air!), its creators now confirm[3], although in light of the limits suggested by the meta-study I referred to earlier the numbers were cautious, but not too bad.

As I just mentioned, the rules for men used to be 21

---

[3] "... According to Richard Smith, a former editor of the British Medical Journal, the level for safe drinking was "plucked out of the air". He was on a Royal College of Physicians team that helped produce the guidelines in 1987. He told *The Times* newspaper that the committee's epidemiologist had conceded that there was no data about safe limits available and that "it's impossible to say what's safe and what isn't". Smith said the drinking limits were "not based on any firm evidence at all", but were an "intelligent guess ...".

Article written by Dr Malcolm Kendrick in *The Independent* Monday 06 April 2015 units per week, with two drink-free days, although the drink-free days were never as high up on the agenda as the units. The UK Government has just reviewed the recommended levels "in light of recent research" and has lowered the 'safe' limits for men down to 14 units per week – exactly the same level as women, with an unclear suggestion that these units should be spread over "3 days or more" with "several drink-free days each week". In the media coverage of the new rules, the lack of clarity in drink-free days has been completely overshadowed by the unit reduction

Personally, I think the new guidelines are unhelpful – on both amount and frequency – certainly for men. Men are at much higher risk from drinking-related problems as we know, so could do with being properly guided, rather than patronised, as some people feel these new guidelines are doing. The evidence from the *JAMA* meta study quoted earlier is quite clear that men have a higher tolerance for alcohol, and that lower mortality was consistent with higher levels of moderate drinking in men (three "drinks" per day vs. two for women). Men are, on average 20% heavier than women (84Kg vs. 70Kg), and this must play a part in the greater tolerance to alcohol observed – both clinically by the scientists at least at moderate levels of drinking – and anecdotally by most of us in real life.

I think most male drinkers will therefore look at these new guidelines of just 14 units per week, and dismiss them out of hand because of this false equivalence.

This then will lead to many people ignoring the rather vague message about taking a few nights off each week as well. Which is the real pity here, because this should have been the real win for the Government to aim for. Giving your liver a regular, weekly break from alcohol must be the best thing you can do to improve your long-term health prospects. My own suggestion, in *The Life of Riley* habits, is for four nights per week abstinence, so I'm being even tougher here than the Government.

I think my approach is healthier, and easier to stick to despite being tougher, because it is designed to be a regular, daily weekday habit. But two days would be better than none, and if the Government had only done that, heavily stressing their existing two day per week break, whilst leaving the overall levels the same, I think most people would have understood that message, and some would have even implemented it. Instead any message about "several drink-free days" will be drowned out by the unit reduction fuss.

Personally I think I would have suggested at least two days not drinking each week (and why not just implant dry Monday/dry Tuesday as a concept), and then over the remaining five days in total suggest 10 to 15 units for women, and 15 to 20 units for men. I'd perhaps also have suggested people target the lower end of the range if they are smaller than average, and the higher end if they are bigger than average. Spread over 5 days this would have been 2-3 units for women, and 3-4 units for men. That's probably too close to the old recommendations of course – and would have looked like the government was doing nothing in the face of increasing concerns over alcohol intake (whether those concerns are well-founded or not).

I wonder too if the government is secretly engaging in a bit of "double-bluffing". They know we'll ignore the recommendations and think it safe to exceed them, so they make the levels extremely low in order to make our view of "excess" lower as well. Who knows?

I really do think the UK Government has scored an own-goal with this advice. I think the target for alcohol consumption within *The Life of Riley* plan as a whole needs to avoid units or quantities altogether. Instead the key here should simply be the goal of becoming a moderate drinker, and I think the best measure for this is your number of nights off:

Target 2 – Don't drink for four nights a week

OK – but what about the weekend, especially once you are into the maintenance element of *The Life of Riley* habits. If you are only drinking three nights per week, how many units is it safe to consume? Taking something that should be spread out over five or seven days, and cramming it into three days, doesn't seem sensible either.

Having tried to make sense of all of the, sometimes heavily conflicting, advice, my view is that once you are comfortably following the habits during the week, and at or around your target weight, I simply can't believe you are putting yourself at significant risk if, as a man, you raise your own per night limits on Friday-Sunday to around six to seven units a night, which is a couple of medium to large glasses of wine, or three pints depending on beer strength, or a bottle of wine split between two people, with a little less for women (maybe four to five units). Over three days, that's 12-15 units for women and 18-21 for men – in line with the old UK government guidelines and still comfortably below the overall weekly units suggested by the *JAMA* study as being associated with reduced mortality, and that's without any of the "wiggle room" created by self-reporting being consistently low. But it's your call.

The six to seven units suggested above is higher, for men at least, than the per night limits currently being recommended, but you would only be consuming alcohol for three nights, and I don't think I know many people who could stick to "just one" on a night where they are drinking. This would still mean across the week you were around (or below) those "risk" marker levels from Dr Porter, and in line with the research on moderate levels being associated with reduced mortality (including the Caerphilly study referenced at the start of this book).

In the end, you must decide for yourself how much you want to drink, but I think the key test of being a moderate drinker is not drinking Monday to Thursday, with the following add-on elements:

- Don't feel guilty about moderate intake overall – it seems to be mildly beneficial;
- Drink sensibly on the two/three nights you do, to keep your weekly count in the safe range;
- Don't regularly engage in "high-risk" binge-drinking. I know many of us will do it once in a while – just don't make it a thing.

So jump on the wagon, even if it's only on school nights.

Chapter 11

"Do the walk of Life"

Walk of Life - Mark Knopfler

Tribe 4 (the sedentary) is the largest single Tribe for a good reason. Lots of people simply hate exercise. Any plan is therefore going to have to work hard to sell this particular aspect of what needs to be done to live longer to a sceptical audience.

And hatred of exercise in all its forms is only one element of the scepticism. Many people have been led to believe that only exercise can help lose weight, and therefore partake under sufferance in order to shed a few lbs. When the weight loss fails to materialise, the hatred of exercise must increase exponentially. This failure is inevitable – unless you are a professional sportsman you simply aren't going to do enough exercise to seriously cut into your daily calorific requirements – and when you do exercise, your brain almost wills you to eat more food "to compensate". Losing weight is not the reason to exercise. Getting fit and physically active, in order to live longer and healthier, is the real reason.

And for those among us who think that the only way to get physically active is to join a gym, sign up for the local half-marathon, or spend thousands of pounds on a bike (and associated lycra) my suggestion that walking for 30 minutes 4 days a week in *The Life of Riley* habits is all you need to get you fit might be greeted with a raised eyebrow. It's almost sacrilegious to suggest something that easy is all that's required.

And I must admit I was sceptical too when I first read about the health benefits of this simple activity. But it's true. Walking really does make a huge difference to fitness.

Now, to be clear, when I say "go for a 30 minute walk" I do not mean a stroll around the shops looking in the windows from time to time. I mean a genuine, properly paced brisk walk that feels as though you are making some effort.

Those of you who are way ahead of this on the fitness stakes can skip this next bit – but for those who have never exercised, here is the plan.

- Make 30 minutes of time in your day – genuinely I suggest doing this at lunchtime, (although I appreciate that won't work for some people, so a different time still works) as you are missing that meal it gives you another focus for your mid-day break, and unlike running or gym work, walking doesn't seem to trigger real hunger pangs, or make you "sweaty" and in need of a shower. I suspect the absence of hunger while walking goes back to the evolutionary principles I discussed earlier. If our ancestors were out walking for a few hours most days hunting for food, feeling ravenous whilst they were doing that would have been massively inconvenient – hence the evolutionary benefit of the lack of pangs.
- For that 30 minutes put on a pair of trainers and leave your office/house/factory.
- Take your smartphone, with a free downloadable app such as Strava or mapmyrun, switch on the app and walk purposefully for 15 minutes (if you can, or start at just 10 if 15 feels too long, or even just 5 if this is really uncharted territory).
- Then turn around and walk purposefully back.

- Normally I'd suggest exercise should be done with friends – it makes for a more enjoyable, motivated experience. But with this I wouldn't necessarily recommend it. Walking with someone leads naturally to chatting, and you will slow down to the pace of the slowest walker – which might, or might not, be you. If you can find someone as keen as you who is prepared to keep up the pace, then great, but please don't let this focused exercise deteriorate into a leisurely stroll/chat with pals. It's too important for you to not get this right.

Instead, why not make a point of doing this regular lunchtime walk alone, and make this a great 30 minute opportunity for reflection on the day, plan for the evening and tomorrow etc. or listen to a podcast, or the radio, or music – but walk purposefully.

Your goal should be to aim to walk out for 15 minutes, and then back for 15 minutes, and for you to complete 2 miles during this 30-minute stretch. That will take some doing if you have never done serious walking before, and it's genuinely not a pace that suits chatting and gazing at the scenery. It is easily doable over time, but you should feel warm, glowing, and possibly slightly out of breath at the end.

If you are just starting out, you need to keep track of progress – this is why those apps are so good, as they will store your walk each day, so you can see over time how you are improving.

I normally finish my walk with a treat – a cappuccino from the local coffee shop before heading back into the office.

I'm then pretty fired up for the afternoon. I don't feel hungry, and the warm liquid fills me up to a degree anyway, and I feel quite smug having done a good 30 minutes.

Do this four times a week and you can claim to be physically active – and qualify for Tribe 5 living longer status.

And that's it – no lycra; bikes; marathon training; gym membership; swimming hassles. Just 4 good 30 minute walks each week, built into your normal routine.

Now 4 x 30 minutes is 120 minutes. UK Government advice is currently 150 minutes of moderate activity a week, but the research evidence suggests 120 is perfectly adequate. And I guarantee once you are into this routine, you will want to extend it. I now walk virtually everywhere I can. I travel to work by train, and get off 20 minutes walk away. If I'm in London, I'll aim to catch an earlier train and will walk virtually wherever I can in the city.

Having a dog helps too. They certainly turn this into a seven day a week habit.

As an observation, most people don't walk fast enough. I'm rarely overtaken when I've been walking through a city (either Birmingham or London – the two I visit most frequently, although NYC is a different matter). If you are a regular walker in and around your town – can I urge you to walk a little faster – not for me but for you. The average speed of urban walking is less than 3 miles per hour (mph), and the health benefits for middle-aged adults of moving up to 3.5 mph or even 4 mph are tremendous. You might expect to slow down a bit from this 4 mph target if you are older, but the evidence supports keeping going as fast as you can, even for people in their 70s and 80s. This was demonstrated by the results of one large-scale USA study[lxxi], which showed that those 70+ adults who walked at a pace faster than 3 mph had a 50% lower risk of coronary heart disease compared to those who walked at less than 2 mph.

And how much benefit does 120 minutes of walking get you?

First, let me define the internationally recognised measure of physical effort, known as a MET (Metabolic Equivalent of a Task). Put simply, this is how much harder something is than effectively doing nothing (sitting on a chair for example). So the effort involved in sitting would rank as a MET of 1, and everything else is ranked by how much more effort it is (or how much energy your body needs to consume to perform it). By the way – this 1 measure is a bit misleading – watching 10 hours of TV a week does not equal 10 METs – you only start to collect them at intensity above 1!

I think we should rework the MET acronym, and make it "Measure of Exercise Toughness" as that is really what it is indicating to us.

When scientists analyse physical activity in this way they are looking at levels of activity that move you beyond normal pottering around, and they measure this in terms of METs expended per hour.

So something really energetic, such as hard running, might clock up 10 METs if you keep it up for an hour. Mowing the lawn for an hour might clock up 5 METs (not if you are on a sit-on of course). Slowly ambling around for an hour might only clock up 2 METs.

Obviously if you perform these activities for less than an hour the number of METs you generate is reduced, and vice versa if you are doing them for longer – or more importantly, repeating them numerous times per week.

And when you add up all these METs, what does it tell us? Well this is a graph published by Harvard[lxxii] on the return on life expectancy from various amounts of exercise.

The X scale on the bottom refers to MET hours/week, so it means the total number of METs you create by partaking in exercise. As a very rough approximation, an hour of walking at 3mph equals 3 METs, and an hour of walking at 4 mph equals 5 METs. So two hours of walking at 3 mph would generate 6 METs, and the same amount of time walking at 4 mph means you are doing 10 MET hours per week.

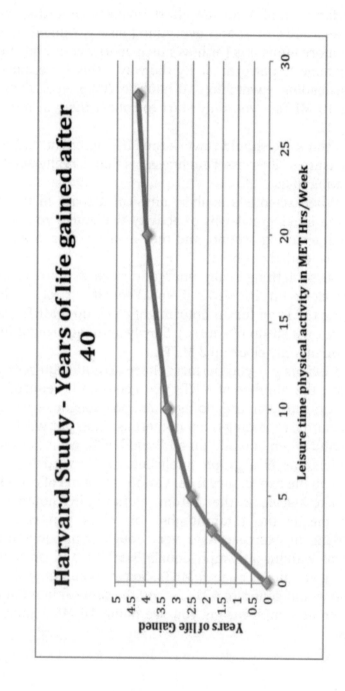

Harvard Study - Years of life gained after 40

Years of life Gained

Leisure time physical activity in MET Hrs/Week

As you can see from the graph, 10 MET's gets you almost 3.5 extra years of life! So 10 METs seems to me to be the perfect final target for the plan.

Target 3 – 10 METs per week

That's one of the reasons I suggest you walk alone, and take a smartphone with you to accurately measure distance and speed. Doing just three mph means you'd only clock up six METs from Monday to Thursday. As you can see from the graph, although the biggest benefit is moving from zero METs to five METs – moving from five METs to ten METs still creates an enormous improvement in life expectancy – so walking faster really can help.

However, trying to add another year extra to your life means moving from around 10 METs to around 25 METs. That's quite a jump, and you can see how the incremental returns start to diminish pretty quickly after about 10 METs.

I actually think that, once you have embraced the walking, you will find yourself sticking other physical activities into your lifestyle, but I have conservatively modelled Tribe 5 on an extra 3.5 years of life, which is around 10 METs per week.

A large study in Norway on men already in their 70s showed that upping the number of 30 minute sessions to 6 per week resulted in 5 extra years of life compared to remaining sedentary[lxxiii] so it is worth trying to do a little more if you can, even as you get older.

In Appendix 1 you can see how many METs you can clock up with a variety of different activities.

If exercise is part of your life already, this chapter will have been a breeze. But if exercise is not your thing, just stick to the walking and aim for that 10 METs per week. But get a move on.

Chapter 12

"Life's what you make it"

Life's what you make it - Talk Talk

Volatility in life expectancy is all around us, and is caused by different variables, and the two key factors which appear to play the biggest part in our odds of longevity are genetics and environment (which in the Western world, given we live in a relatively benign environment, is strongly influenced individually by our lifestyle and wealth/class). Which of these factors – genetic or environment has the biggest effect?

Just for the moment, I'm going to leave the issue of whether your social class determines your lifestyle and just work on lifestyle factors (the five Tribes) vs. genetics, and will come back to socioeconomic factors later.

I hear people say life expectancy is all in the genes – and that because our genetic make-up is outside our control, it's not worth over-worrying about our lifestyle and the environment we create for ourselves.

Well, there's some truth to that of course, but not nearly as much as the fatalists would have you believe.

Of course there are genetic differences between all of us, and these differences, along with both blind luck and our lifestyle choices, affect our longevity. I've been describing population effects in this book – but you will know of "blameless" friends and relatives tragically lost early due to cancer or stroke. By the same token, you will have people close to you living blissfully into their 90s without ever being aware that they were paragons of virtue, and of course we are all aware of the (apocryphal?) tales of our best mate's

"Uncle Tommy" who smoked and drank until he was 103! Helmut Schmidt, the former Chancellor of Germany, died aged 96. He was a 60 per day chain-smoker, and apparently hoarded 10,000s of menthol cigarettes at his home in case they were made illegal. He apparently quit cold-turkey in September 2015 after an operation. He died in November! So these characters do exist. And of course at the level of the individual there is luck, blind chance, pre-disposition, call it what you will.

And by the way – "blameless" is a poor word. I don't blame anyone for choosing to live in a particular way – our bodies are our own to do with as we see fit in my view. If you want to smoke, or drink, or be overweight or sedentary – that's your choice to make. I only hope it's a properly informed choice, which is part of the reason I wrote this book.

But I would argue that at a population level, genetics seems to have a smaller variability effect than the lifestyle choices that create your own personal "environment".

Of course your inherited genetic make-up is the starting point for life expectancy. Interestingly though, unless you come from a line of long-lived folk it's probably difficult to tell your likely genetic make-up in this regard, because so many of our ancestors who passed on young will have done so because of medical conditions which can now be cured, or lifestyle causes you were only dimly aware of, or even hazardous working conditions pretty much eliminated from modern society. So despite dying young, your ancestors might not have been carrying and transmitting "poor genetic stock", so you can't necessarily predict your own longevity because of their age of passing.

Of course a few people will know they carry some likelihood for illness due to genetics, and these days will be given advice on how to try to counteract this. For most of us though, our genes are the cards we've been given in the game of life, and for good or ill we need to cope with what we've got, even if we don't quite know how good a hand we've been dealt.

And, in order to separate the effects of genes and environment (in which I for now include both class and our lifestyle choices as a single alternative factor) let me pose a thought experiment. Imagine a perfect world. No tobacco, people only drank moderately, everyone was a healthy weight and ate well, and we all took care of our bodies by exercising to a reasonable degree. We would all still have different life expectancies of course, but the evidence suggests that if we all had a "live longer Tribe 5" lifestyle our average (mean) life expectancy as a population today would be up in the late 80s/low 90s, and deaths would be tightly clustered around that age, with around two thirds of us dying within 7 years or so either side of this age. And that spread from early 80s to late 90s for most people would be influenced by social status, genetic make-up, and of course a bit of blind luck. There would be outliers too of course. Your genetic history (or luck or social status) might pre-dispose you to an early grave, or a telegram from the Queen, but in all likelihood we would mostly be crowding around that early 80s to late 90s age range.

Now in the Five Tribes model, Tribe 1 (the heavy drinkers) based on the German study have an average (mean) life expectancy of 59, with two thirds of these alcohol dependent folk dying between the ages of 48 and 70. Of course a few are dying even younger, and some are hanging on into their 70s (and possibly beyond). Tribes 2 and 3 similarly start their upward curve quite early.

And what does this tell us about the effect of genetics vs. lifestyle. Well, we know the model is a reasonably accurate indicator of real life, because the two graphs look so similar. So compared to my thought experiment, we know that the overall range of human death starts in earnest with some of our heavy drinkers, as young as 47 for men, and starts to curve upwards for people in their 50s and 60s quite quickly. So because of lifestyle factors, the population-wide adult human life-span is over 50 years – yet the genetic/ /blind luck baseline span for most people could (and arguably should) be as little as 14 years.

So genes play some part – but arguably these days the lifestyle you choose (and/or your social class) is much more important overall.

Social Class vs. Lifestyle

The other factor outside of our control to a degree is of course our relative wealth/class/socio-economic status. It's well known that life expectancy for someone living in the east end of Glasgow is considerably lower than someone living in the leafy suburbs of Esher in Surrey.

And of course I started this whole project after the deaths of three colleagues who, because of their occupation, were paid-up members of the middle classes. So my trigger here wasn't to point out the health consequences of social injustice, even though there clearly are some.

Access to good quality health-care (both NHS and private health-care of course playing a part), riskier/harder working conditions, a general level of education exposing you to positive health messages – these factors are all bound to play a role in that yawning gap in life expectancy.

However, also playing a large role is the relative frequency of poor lifestyle choices within the different socio-demographic classes. In one major study by the Department of Epidemiology and Public Health, University College London[lxxiv] into both behaviours and attitudes towards health, factored by class, they confirmed that smoking rates are much higher for those in the lower two socioeconomic bands (DEs) than the two highest bands (ABs), at a ratio of about 2.5 to 1. Similarly the AB classes were twice as likely to partake in exercise, and eat healthily.

The ABs also felt more in control of their health, and

perceived themselves more likely to live longer – certainly feeling much more likely to live into their 80s. DEs were much less likely to think long-term or about their future health and what they could be doing to stay healthy, although there was a much smaller gap between the ABs and DEs in how much they thought about future illnesses (confirming my earlier comment that we are all guilty of self-denial when we choose to be).

There are lots of other studies confirming this 'healthy' bias amongst the top socioeconomic classes as far as smoking and exercise is concerned, although there is less of a bias with other lifestyle factors.

As far as obesity is concerned, there is a direct link with income for women. According to the NHS NOO in 2012[lxxv], 31% of the bottom fifth of women by income are obese, but only 19% of the top fifth by income. Interestingly for men there is no real split, with equivalent figures of 25% for the bottom fifth, and 24% for the top fifth.

And finally, the fourth horseman of my apocalypse, drinking too much, is of course much more of a "middle class" lifestyle trend, as evidenced by this report from the HSCIC[lxxvi].

So what percentage of adverse health outcomes is due to the environment poorer people find themselves in (access to worse jobs, shops, health and educational facilities etc.), and what percentage is simply due to people in those environments on balance (but not exclusively) making bad lifestyle choices? I'm loath to venture too far into this issue for fear of straying into complex political waters. However, a team of researchers at The University of York did some interesting analysis that would support my view, and the main thrust of the argument in this book, that it is lifestyle choices, not socioeconomic class, which are the main determinants of life expectancy.[lxxvii]

What I will say is while I think it is difficult for people to shift en-masse in terms of class, social background, economic circumstances etc., it is possible to shift in terms of lifestyle. Living in poverty does not mean you have to smoke. Nor does it mean you are forced to drink heavily. Neither does it mean you cannot take the simple steps required to become physically active (particularly walking).

The one area where there is legitimate cause for dispute might be healthy eating. Some deprived parts of the UK are quite accurately described as "food deserts' where there are no household name supermarkets, just poorly stocked convenience stores and a surfeit of fast-food outlets. However, I'm not sure the five 'Life of Riley' habits are beyond all but the very poorest. Porridge with milk for breakfast should cost less than 40p per serving, and I think the sort of meals I describe in Appendix 3 (if you were preparing four dinners per week for two people) ought not to cost more than £5 per head. But that means you need the £40 to start with for those four nights, and you need ready access to shops that sell the sorts of ingredients required to make those meals. More of a challenge for the most deprived I accept – and as I said before, perhaps this is a political/social problem outside the scope of this book. It is interesting though to note that despite not living in food deserts, the most well-off men had obesity rates equivalent to the least well-off. Another book I suspect!

But for the vast majority of people, no matter their social status, lifestyle choices are for them individually to make, and whether you live in the east end or Esher, the right choices will add years to your life. A recent study (commissioned by the electronics company Phillips to promote some health equipment, but still interesting) said this view was in tune with most of us. 87% of us said individuals should take responsibility for their health, a view backed up by 94% of doctors they surveyed.

In the end, there's little you can do about poor luck leading to accidents or early illness onset. And there's virtually nothing you can do about your genes (yet – but scientists are working on it). And it's arguable whether or not you can change your social class (although many do of course).

But the one thing you can do is to increase your average life expectancy by getting into the "live longer Tribe 5", where whatever your genetic or social background, your genes are working against an average life expectancy of 90, rather than Tribes 1-4, where your genes and social class are impacting a potentially much lower age of death.

Chapter 13

"I hope I die before I get old"

My Generation – The Who

"In the end, it's not the years in your life that count. It's the life in your years."

Abraham Lincoln

When I've been talking to people about this book, and the concept of *The Life of Riley* habits, one recurring theme crops up, which is the argument "I don't want to live anther five years if it's going to be in a care home or in and out of hospital". In fact, as I referred to earlier, one recent study said that, if given the choice, people would rather live a shorter life than a long one if they could be guaranteed their health to the end of their lives[lxxviii]. This study was a well-intentioned effort to raise the issue of poor end-of-life care – one well worth doing. But the choice being proffered (health vs. lifespan) isn't what is on offer in real life. I can clearly see why people would make that argument or pick that choice if it could somehow be open to them. But it's completely fallacious, for two reasons

First, as I touched on earlier, we are all going to be "inconvenienced" to a degree at the end of life – going to the doctors more often, going to hospital, maybe even needing permanent care and support. But that is true of the last few years before we shuffle off, no matter what age that might be. And you will recall my argument that those folk living later due to better lifestyle will also suffer fewer years of inconvenience. So, remembering my splitting the life expectancy tables in half from earlier, if the years from age

65 onwards are a bit grim for someone eventually dying at 75, so too potentially will the years from age 84 be for someone shuffling off at 90. But they will have had good health from 65 to 84 – almost 20 years more.

This is a key benefit of the plan. You don't "lose out" by living longer. You'll only have the same, if not fewer, years of inconvenience. The extra years are all "good years".

And second, those "good years" are likely to be spent in even better health if you are following a lifestyle like *The Life of Riley* habits, because the other huge benefit from the exercising element (simple as it is) is that it will make you fitter, and your later years more enjoyable, and your years of "inconvenience" are also likely to be shorter and, well, less "inconvenient".

Let's be clear, according to the (admittedly simplistic) 5 Tribes model, around 70% of those people dying before they are 80 will be in Tribes 1-3, and their later years are likely to involve trips to hospital, serious illness of some form or other, or general infirmity. Conversely, over three quarters of those dying past 85 will be in Tribes 4 and 5. Now I'm not saying they will all die peacefully in their sleep, but all the evidence suggests their passing is likely to be less traumatic, shorter at its end, and more in their control.

And what does the evidence say about the qualitative benefits of being in Tribe 5? Let's sell in another key benefit of the plan right here as "staying younger longer". This of course has been the key benefit extolled by beauty cream manufacturers for decades, but the reality is that it would seem that moderate exercise is the real key here to staying younger longer, rather than fancy chemicals in a white cream.

The habits focus on walking, but a study of older cyclists (which I'd argue is the next step up from walking as you get on in life) found some remarkable benefits. This study was conducted by a team of researchers from Kings College in London[lxxix]. The researchers picked 120 fit cyclists

(80 men and 40 women) at a range of ages from 55 to 79, and tested them across a range of physical functions commonly associated with deterioration over time as you age – things like aerobic fitness, resting heart rate, muscle density, skeletal mass and breathing ability.

They were looking to see how much these facilities diminished as the cyclists got older.

These riders had to be reasonably proficient on a bike – capable of riding 60 miles in 6.5 hours for the men (so about 9.5 mph) and 40 miles in 5.5 hours for the women (so about 7 mph). I don't know anyone who puts on lycra who wouldn't think that was a pretty straightforward task, and I'd hazard a guess that if you were a regular brisk walker, you could transfer to that level of cycling pretty easily if you wanted to – so we are not talking about supermen or women here. They also excluded heavy drinkers and smokers (not many cyclists smoke in my experience, and although a post-ride beer or glass of wine is almost de rigeur, I wouldn't think we'd need to exclude too many on the grounds of alcohol dependency).

The cyclists underwent two days of intense laboratory testing at King's. Researchers tested reflexes, muscle strength, oxygen uptake along with peak explosive cycling power, and a whole range of metabolic and endocrine functions, along with general health and well-being measures.

After analysing the results, the scientists were amazed to discover they could hardly tell the older riders apart from the younger ones.

The data showed that the effects of getting older were far from obvious, and the lead scientist, Professor Stephen Harridge, quoted in *The Times* said *"It is not ageing itself which brings about poor function and frailty, but the fact that people have stopped exercising and are no longer active"*.

In one basic test, which involved standing up from a chair, walking three metres and then sitting down again, the oldest participants were well within the scores recorded by healthy young adults.

Although the researchers chose cycling, they are convinced most other forms of aerobic activity would yield similar outcomes.

I'm 56 now, and consider myself in pretty good shape – certainly capable of performing demanding physical exercise and capable of managing most tasks. To think I might still feel pretty much this good aged 79 or 80 is fantastic – and certainly motivation for me to get back on my bike as soon as possible.

And being active until you are 90 is a real possibility too. One study[lxxx] tracked almost 2,500 healthy men from their 70s onwards. The 41% who were still alive 20 years later were much more likely to be non-smokers who exercised and managed their weight, and these survivors had significantly better late-life physical function and mental well-being, with over two thirds of these survivors rating their late-life health as excellent or very good.

So another key benefit of sticking with *The Life of Riley* habits is that it will make you feel younger and healthier well into old age.

This is one of the many really encouraging pieces of research which confirms the basic premise behind *The Life of Riley* habits, that making a few basic changes now can have dramatically beneficial effects later (not least of which is still being alive of course!)

Only recently I was cycling up to the Col de sa Batalla in the Tramuntana Mountains in Mallorca. This is one of my favourite climbs – a lung-busting 35 minutes in the lowest gear you can find, climbing a gradient of around 5% for 8 Km. About half way up, I overtook an older guy on a pretty snazzy bike. Saying hi to him, I recognised a cycling top local to me, and I was given a good dose of Brummie humour as I cycled past (no one likes being overtaken on a climb!) At the top there's a café, and he came up to me to chat when he arrived. He was a stalwart of the Solihull Cycling Club (famous in the Midlands) and was 80 years old. He'd been cycling all his life. When I try to compare the challenge he had just completed with the state of health of my mum, who was almost exactly the same age as this chap, but who had died two years earlier – well there is no comparison.

If I can still climb Sa Batalla when I am 80 I will be a happy man.

Chapter 14

"I may be losing my mind"

Losing My Mind – Maroon 5

It's all very well me banging on about you getting into Tribe 5, and living into your 90s or beyond – but if you end up suffering from Alzheimer's or one of the other conditions collectively known as dementia, those latter years might not be much fun, either for you, your partner or the rest of your family. One in six people over 80 have dementia so it is a major concern for us as a society as we continue to age.

So let's turn that number around and start with the very good news – the vast majority of people do not get dementia. And there are very good reasons to think that sticking to *The Life of Riley* habits can improve your chances of remaining alert and aware all through your life.

There is no cure for dementia. Alzheimer's in particular has been stubbornly resistant to the best efforts of the research community, although of late some researchers at Duke University have discovered some new methods of slowing down the disease (in mice, again)[lxxxi].

But given there is no cure as yet, prevention is the key. The good news is that many of *The Life of Riley* habits – eating healthily, being fit, and not being alcohol dependent, are associated with lower levels of dementia.

Dr Doug Brown, director of research and development at The Alzheimer's Society, was recently quoted in *The Guardian*[lxxxii] as saying *"the four key evidence-based strategies for preventing dementia are exercise, not smoking, a healthy diet and looking after your heart"*. Great news, as all four of those strategies are at the heart of *The Life of Riley* habits.

It's also worth noting one of the outcomes of the Welsh Study I referred to earlier (The Caerphilly Study). It followed just over 2,500 men over 35 years and found that regular exercise (30 minutes walking five times a week, or equivalent) in adult life is the single most important factor in reducing the risk of dementia. The other factors were important too, but exercising trumped them all.

Similarly a recent study in Finland which followed 1,260 people aged 60-77[lxxxiii], and effectively split them into two groups, showed at the end of two years, that those who had been eating a better diet (they were on a traditional Finnish diet, with oily fish twice a week), getting exercise (they did dancing, but I'm sure purposeful walking would have the same effect) and training their brains (they used computerised games, but again Sudoku etc. will work as well) scored on average 25% higher in mental tests than those in the other group. Now this wasn't specifically looking at dementia, but its potential precursor, declines in mental function. These results were in part replicated recently by a study for The Alzheimer's Society, run by King's College, which also showed computerised/online games helped mental functioning in older people[lxxxiv].

Finally a huge study on over 20,000 older women in the USA conducted by researchers from Harvard[lxxxv] found significant positive correlation between maintaining physical activity and higher cognitive function. They particularly pointed out the benefits of walking *"...which indicated significant associations between better cognitive performance and 5.2 or more MET-hours/wk of energy expenditure..."*.

However, in a major piece of research that shocked the scientists concerned, obesity (and to a lesser extent being overweight) was associated with lower levels of dementia[lxxxvi]. As this was a meta-study of almost two million people it represents the most striking piece of analysis ever done on this subject. It seems the beneficial effects increased in proportion to the level of obesity of the individual concerned.

Some scientists are questioning the results, stating the very long time periods involved, the difficulty in getting an accurate diagnosis of dementia, and the tendency for those with dementia to become thinner and reduce their BMI having the effect of skewing the data, but nevertheless, the survey was striking in its conclusion.

Now you might be thinking, what's the point of me losing weight if it means I'm going to put myself at higher risk of losing my faculties? Well, I actually think this research is a really good piece of news, for the following reason:

I simply can't see a logical reason why the correlation between obesity and lower levels of dementia is lifestyle related, i.e. I can't think of something overweight people are actively doing at a lifestyle level that would cause lower dementia levels (I'm not being facetious when I say this – but there's no evidence the overweight are doing more crossword puzzles etc.).

Therefore if it is not lifestyle-related, but it is directly proportional to weight gain, then it is highly likely that being overweight or obese implies something is happening within that person's body which is having the unplanned side effect of causing lower dementia. And this is likely to be a chemical or physical change within the body. And if it is, scientists should be able to find that change. And once they do, they may well have found a treatment or cure for the disease. And one that can hopefully be administered without the side effects of carrying too much weight.

One theory is that Alzheimer's is actually "type 3 diabetes" because it is potentially the effect of sugar on the brain that causes this disease, and that people who are obese are "good" at packing sugar away into fat cells, meaning less gets into the brain, thereby meaning less dementia[lxxxvii]. If that is the case, taking in less sugar to begin with would be a really good plan, which of course is hard-wired into the five habits.

In the meantime, there are other things you can do too.

There's increasing evidence that keeping your mind active helps enormously. Anecdotal evidence points to crosswords, Sudoku, Kenken and other brainteaser type activity, but there is much more work to do here. What is certain is an active, enquiring mind is paramount.

If the general odds of getting dementia are one in six, and nearly all of the things within *The Life of Riley* habits are associated with lowering your chances of getting the disease, then there really is relatively little to worry about if you are following the plan. Not a bad benefit to end on.

Chapter 15

"People stay, just a little bit longer"

Stay - Jackson Browne

You may have heard of a business concept known as 'continuous improvement". This actually started life in Japan after the second world war, where it is called Kaizen. The great thing about Kaizen is it can be applied across all fields of human endeavour, and is equally seen at work in science these days. The rate of scientific progress across all fields of human endeavour over the last fifty years has been simply amazing. Some of this has of course been due to break-through technological and scientific developments, but much of it has also been due to slow, incremental improvements in lots of areas of health and medicine.

We might not notice it much on a day-to-day basis, but going back to the mid-60s and comparing life then to today is profoundly uplifting.

Computing had barely begun to creep into general life – and then only via giant machines hermetically sealed off from human contact. Even in the 70s, when I did my bachelors degree in computer studies, most of our time was spent gazing through glass windows at giant tape machines whirring away and banks of flashing lights. Today we all have more powerful computers sitting in our pockets as smartphones.

50 years ago, if you wanted to know about things, you either needed to have been well educated, spend a lot of time at your local library, or have access to an Encyclopaedia Britannica (or similar). Today, the entire world is available

at our fingertips via the internet and search engines.

In my own business, broadcasting, we've gone from 3 black and white analogue TV channels to 1000s of digital stations from around the world, with more online, and DVDs containing the most extraordinary visual content. And radio too has gone through a transformation, from pirates on medium wave, to hundreds of digital stations, and 1000s of online services and podcasts available from around the world.

These are all terrific advances – but perhaps they pale in comparison to some of the biggest progress being made, namely in the world of medicine and life sciences. Smarter surgical techniques, better drugs, improved scanning, imaging and diagnosis have all helped to dramatically improve life expectancy.

In fact, in the UK, average (median) life expectancy for mature adults (i.e. excluding the influence of those dying under 30) has increased from 77 to 84 since 1980 – a boost of 7 years in just 3 decades. Men have seen a faster increase over this period – a growth of 8 years from 74 to 82. Women, who were much more likely to live longer to begin with, have seen a slower increase in the median age of life expectancy, but still by an impressive 5 years, from 81 to 86.

Perhaps the most intriguing element of this shift is that it is occurring across all boundaries.

You might reasonably expect that advances in medicine would help those who become ill or sick younger, and that is certainly the case. The median life expectancy for the bottom quintile (i.e. the 20% who died youngest) in 1980-82 was just 54 in men, and 60 in women. Over the past 30 years this has risen dramatically. The youngest 20% to die now have a median life expectancy of 61 for men and 67 for women – so progress of just over 7 years in life for both sexes in just 30 years for those most at risk.

But the encouraging thing for me (and this book) is the continuing growth in median life expectancy for the oldest 20% – those who survive the longest. 30 years ago, this age was 87 for men and 92 for women. Today it's 93 and 96; so over 6 years improvement for men, and 4 years for women.

So medical advances are boosting the life expectancy of those at the bottom end of the graph, and those at the top – and although the increases are bigger at the bottom, as you'd expect, even at the top end of the scale they are pretty impressive. Some improvements will also be due to changing lifestyles, with reductions in smoking levels being the obvious factor – although the rise in obesity might serve to negate much of the positive effects due to the decline in smoking. I suspect this is a whole new area for some comparative research.

If you take the oldest 20% as a decent proxy for Tribe 5 it means that we can expect people in Tribe 5 to live even longer in the future – if medical advances continue.

And here I am going to dive into the unknown and suggest that all the evidence points to continuing progress. That Lancet study from the UK Medical Research Council I mentioned in Chapter 3 suggests that mean life expectancy overall for the UK will grow by around 6 years for men and 4 years for women _in the next 15 years_ due to a combination of factors – that's twice as fast as recent trends, although they didn't spilt this out by top and bottom quintiles, and it's mean rather than median which might be expected to grow slightly faster.

I hope the researchers are right in their forecast of rapidly increasing life expectancy across the board, because then my figures are under-playing the great boost for us just around the corner.

And the UK Government's own statistics are also highly positive for life expectancy extensions. The latest ONS data[lxxxviii] forecasts suggest that over the next 25 years mean life expectancy will increase by 5 years overall, and by up to

8 years over the next 50. Again, this is for everyone, so not split out by top and bottom, but as we now know those differences aren't huge.

And what might be driving this continued growth, across all Tribes. Three main factors seem to be exciting most scientists.

1 – Big data and personal computing

This is really two inter-linked points.

First, the rise of smart-phones, wearable devices etc. is providing us with access to far more information about our own health than ever before. The number of people wearing fitbits or other tracking devices is staggering.

My wife regularly chirps "I'm vibrating" whilst we are out walking, with a great sense of pride! My best mate in radio, John Myers, often tweets *"off to do my 10,000 steps"*. Fantastic – being motivated by a computer chip.

Technology is providing us with our own personal trainers. And I think these devices are pretty crude compared to what might be around the corner. Imagine wearing a skin patch that monitored breathing, pulse rate, perspiration levels as well as motion, and wirelessly transmitting that to your smart-phone, and then onwards to some cloud based database that can keep track of your progress and vital signs. All that technology exists today – it's just a question of bringing it all together. One company is already trying to do just that[lxxxix].

Second, you have the benefits of pulling that data together at a macro level. Apple and IBM recently announced a collaboration to allow users of Apple iPhones, smart watches etc. to store that data in the cloud, with IBM able to then anonymously collate and share that information with doctors, researchers etc. Although there are clearly personal data privacy implications here, this move to sharing real data from millions of individuals, rather than relying on small survey numbers, could revolutionise how we measure the effects of fitness and diet changes.

The benefits here don't rely on everyone participating in electronic tracking, but the significant numbers who do will provide a huge database for research.

2 – Smart diagnosis

This ranges from better MRI and ultrasound scanning, which proponents think might allow you to go for a once a year scan, identify changes, and then essentially zap any pre-cancerous tumours spotted, all the way through to being able to use your smartphone (or have your doctor use hers) to self-administer simple diagnostic tests and send them away for immediate analysis. One technique, known as digital diffraction diagnosis (D3) would allow doctors to perform analysis on tissues (such as those obtained during a cervical smear test for example) using simple equipment attached to a smart phone to test for cancers, with the images then sent off for central analysis. The tests can cost as little as £1.20, compared to the £100s/£1,000s it can currently cost.

We are also now seeing new types of blood tests that can pick up cancers years before they become more obvious[xc]. This sort of simple, inexpensive testing can only increase over time, with enormously beneficial results.

3 – Personalised/genetic medicine

This is also developing fast, with DNA therapy having the potential to treat/eliminate many genetic conditions. The NHS recently launched the "100,000 genomes project" as a trial in bringing more tailored treatment and smarter drugs into play, by sampling the genetic make-up of 100,000 people who either had typical cancers and other diseases with a genetic component, along with genetically sampling their relatives. This data is then going to be anonymously shared with drug and research facilities to help develop new cures for these diseases. New genetic-marking techniques for identifying the types of cancerous cells in prostate cancer, for example, are leading to potentially ground-breaking treatments[xci].

There are a host of other improvements coming along too. Here are just a few areas of scientific progress culled from recent headlines.

- Robotic surgery is one example, allowing the work of the best surgeons to be replicated, or allowing all surgeons to work on a much more detailed microscopic level than they have been allowed to before[xcii]. Limited so far, this can only become more useful as computing power increases.
- Immunology replacing chemotherapy as a "miracle" cure for cancer[xciii].
- The use of nanotechnology to repair damage in our bodies at a cellular level[xciv], including the development of stem cell technology to be able to cure Parkinson's/Alzheimers by repairing and regrowing damaged brain tissue[xcv].
- Stem cells will also be used, with other technologies, to grow new organs and tissue. Alongside better materials being discovered every day, this will allow for better prosthetics[xcvi].
- And scientists in the USA are now describing one particular area of research as "senolytics", for a new class of drugs which they hope will slow down the ageing process by getting rid of dead or 'senescent" cells. In research conducted at the Mayo Clinic and reported in *The Guardian*[xcvii], tests on mice (it's always mice) have proved remarkably positive, with the drugs producing improved cardiovascular

function, better stamina, reduced osteoporosis and frailty, and extended healthy lifespan.

In any one week you will see dozens of news reports in the papers on exciting new medical and research developments. The possibilities are endless, and you can see why these technologies will allow the age to which we might live (and live healthily) to keep on growing towards our natural span.

But this growth in life expectancy can't continue ad infinitum. To begin with there's a sensible starting point to take which is you are born with a certain genetic "time clock" inside you, and you are unlikely to live beyond that – with all of the lifestyle factors I have discussed (smoking, drinking, obesity, lack of exercise) simply serving to speed that clock up, and run down your time prematurely.

In addition, most scientists believe that whatever your individual genetic code, overall there is a natural limit to life span, and have suggested a range from 110 to 120. In the view of most experts, all of this advance in medical technology will simply push us closer to that natural limit, and allow us to live healthier lives closer to the end. Not everyone believes this of course, and some on the fringes believe there might be no limit to life span – but as no one has experienced that yet (or at least not scientifically proven) I think I'll stick with the mainstream view.

And what does that mean for you and me – aiming to be healthy members of Tribe 5? Well, it means that even though the median age of Tribe 5 life expectancy is currently 89 for men and 91 for women, this is likely to increase, as we eliminate things which cause our "time clock" to tick faster, and increasingly catch, via medical intervention, the random acts of nature which up until now have taken people "before their time".

Predicting the future is of course notoriously difficult, but three points do stand out as giving some real comfort to any predictions.

- All the scientific research shows that living a Tribe 5 life will significantly boost your chances of being in the top 20% who live the longest.
- Data for that 20% who survive the longest already show median life expectancy today to be almost 95 (higher than my own estimates for Tribe 5).
- All of the evidence suggests medical advances can put years onto these figures for people some age away from those target lifespans.

The ONS have helpfully modelled all of this thinking on the "dynamic" effects of all of this activity on future life expectancy[xcviii]. They have a very simple life expectancy calculator too. It only asks your current age and sex, to produce a single "average" number for you. What is interesting is how this dynamic number varies from the current static average (median), which we know for men and women is 82 and 86 respectively. The ONS modelling suggests typical male life expectancy will improve by around 5 years during an adult lifetime with most adult men now forecast to live on average to 87 or 88, and for women it will improve by around 3 years to 88 or 89.

Although the ONS data isn't split out by Tribes, it's a reasonable assumption to make that the live longer Tribe 5 folk will capture most of these extended years too, pushing likely life expectancy for them up into the low to mid-90s.

For someone in their mid 50s like me, the prospect of being able to live for another 35 years or so is a pretty nice thought to finish on.

Chapter 16

"This is the end"

The End – Doors

I always thought Jim Morrison sounded just like Perry Como – although they certainly dressed differently.

Both of course sang about the great existential truths of our time. We are only alive once, and the end comes to all of us, but we should enjoy life while we are here.

The Doors Magnum Opus, *The End* was of course rather bleak in its outlook. Whilst Jim sang *"This is the end, beautiful friend, this is the end, my only friend, the end "*, Perry's most famous line was much more uplifting, when he sang about *"...magic moments, filled with love."*

When you read great thinkers and eminent philosophers discussing lives well lived, they always seem to come back to the same point. What would be your epitaph? What will people say about you when they gather at your funeral? If they can say you were true friends, and/or that you had magic moments together, filled with love, you've probably done all right.

When I started researching and writing this book, I was thinking a lot about those friends who had died too soon, and about loved ones as well. And the point that struck home most was that if you changed your lifestyle, by just a little, you could easily add 10 or even 15 years to your life. And that's the life of a child – maybe your own grandchild. What a gift, to be able to spend time with your grand-children, in good health, giving them true love and magic moments to remember you by.

Being more selfish I also thought about the now ubiquitous bucket lists we are all supposed to prepare. I'd bet pretty much all of them would have something adventurous on them, or at least strenuous. Something we've put off doing for most of our working lives because of time, money or family constraints. Well it's no good getting to the point where those constraints have been lifted, only to find you're too unwell or unfit to actually do the thing you've spent your life thinking about.

Whatever is on your own bucket list – the last item should surely be the ability to give the list to your grand-kids while on your death-bed, and tell them you ticked everything off so they can write and then read out a glowing obituary to you at your funeral or cremation (I'm going down in flames by the way, to the strains of "Born To Run" by Bruce).

One of my favourite columnists is Melanie Reid of *The Times*. Melanie, you may know, is tetraplegic after breaking her neck and back in a riding accident in April 2010. Her "Spinal Column" appears each Saturday and is worth buying the paper for on its own.

Recently she wrote a very moving piece observing how we are all, generally, moving from calling our middle years being "middle aged" into describing this period as "later youth". Of course she goes on to compare the fabulous luxury we all have in this "later youth" period with her own privations. Not in a mawkish way, because she is too good a writer for that. But reading a tetraplegic discussing the golden opportunities offered to those of us lucky enough to be alive today, with the potential to remain fit, healthy, active and involved late into our 70s, 80s and beyond, was a powerful wake-up call. We can continue to look stylish (well some of us can – others, like me, never got that memo), keep up to date with the latest electronic gadgets and gizmos, travel the world for less money than ever before, and enjoy all the delights of a connected media-abundant society.

She and I are similar ages, and she captured perfectly in the column the changing nature of the generations. Her parents (and mine) were middle-aged to us when kids. They looked different, acted different, and in some ways had moved out of "youth" and into some way-station before old-age as we were growing up. That's just not true of today's generation of 40 and 50 somethings.

Let me quote her most poignant sentence, which struck me to the quick:

"....believe me, if life is the Tour de France, where you are now is a supreme state of grace: a period of incredible lightness of being, when you are no longer chasing, striving, pedalling uphill, but can freewheel, sit up, look at the scenery, enjoy everything around you. Odds are you'll have loads of time until the road starts to slope downhill..."

Melanie was absolutely right to prompt those of us lucky enough to be able to do these things to do them well, and live a fulfilled and good life. And my addendum would simply be, don't squander your health if you don't have to.

The "Life of Riley" habits are only a simple guide, but the idea behind them is universal. We do only get to live once, and the end will come to us all – but you can defer the ultimate graduation ceremony for quite some time if you try just a little bit harder.

Postscript

The art of time management

My favourite management guru, Peter Drucker (who I'm pleased to say lived to the ripe old age of 95), was certainly focussed on managing one's time. It was probably his main focus when coaching executives on effectiveness. Two of his quotes resonate:

"Until we can manage time, we can manage nothing else."

"Everything requires time. It is the only truly universal condition. All work takes place in time and uses up time. Yet most people take for granted this unique, irreplaceable, and necessary resource. Nothing else, perhaps, distinguishes effective executives as much as their tender loving care of time."

I too am a devotee of effective time management. I have given my own staff and managers countless lunchtime time-management seminars over the years. I think it is probably the single most effective discipline you can instil in someone.

And in the course of writing this book, I have come to the rather obvious conclusion that *The Life of Riley* habits are, collectively, nothing more really than a giant exercise in time management. For what is the point of being able to save an hour here, half a day there, trimming and tidying your diary relentlessly, if in the end it's all for naught, and the years you have saved are foolishly cast aside.

I've spent many lunchtimes helping my teams to save minutes and hours.

Here, by following *The Life of Riley* habits I hope to have helped you save years, and even decades.

That truly would be effective time management – something I hope my hero Mr Drucker would be proud of.

The Plan on a page

It's always a useful business exercise to see if you can fit your plan onto a single sheet of A4. People are busy, concentration spans are limited, and so being able to condense your thinking into something that's readable in a minute is very powerful. In that spirit, here is *The Life of Riley* concept – on a page.

Objective:

To significantly improve the odds of people living a much longer, healthier life.

Strategy

- Segment the population into Tribes by lifestyle, and use the evidence to prove there are real life expectancy differences due to those lifestyle choices.
- Create a scientifically sound plan to move people into the right Tribe for greatest life expectancy.
- Create a marketing campaign based on the key benefits to those individuals.

Execution

- Create five simple habits to live by.
- Make the plan as easy to follow as possible to give it "stickability".
- Stick in a phased introduction to give people some early wins.
- Give the habits some flexibility to give people the feeling of control.
- Test it on yourself.

Measurement

- Identify three easy to measure targets/KPIs.
- Moving closer each week towards a "Trethefen" BMI of 22 – 25 (the Big Hairy Arsed Goal).
- Not drinking four nights a week.
- Walking for 30 minutes 4 times a week.

Those Benefits in Full

- By adopting *The Life of Riley* habits you should live up to 15 years longer on average than those who make the worst lifestyle choices. That length of time represents a full generation of extra life.

- Scientific advances mean that could end up being an average life expectancy figure of around 95 for most people, and even 100 if you are still young.

- Your extra years are likely to be all "good" years, and cutting down on your weight and the booze means your "end of life" inconveniences are likely to be shorter and less unpleasant. This means potentially an extra 20 years or more of "healthy living".

- Maintaining physical activity means you will feel younger and healthier for much, much longer.

- You are doing all of the things which science reckons hold back the onset of dementia.

Appendix 1

MET Tables

MET means "Metabolic Equivalent of a Task", or as I have renamed it, "Measurement of Exercise Toughness".

If you look online there are dozens of different sources for METs. None is perfect. True accuracy would depend upon knowing your age, weight, fitness level and the intensity of your workout. But as a rough rule of thumb they are all pretty good. I've picked out an average rating to give you a good guide to each type of exercise.

Just as a reminder, this is a measure of how tough something is, compared to doing nothing. Normally a MET measure is given for doing an hour of something, so if you only do 30 minutes you need to halve the MET score.

Most sport and exercise will give you some METs, but they aren't the only things you can do which are good for you. Other activities which do have a MET score include housework, chores, DIY etc. Worth investigating if that's something you do a lot of, but it's an area of life I have singularly failed to excel at.

And remember, our Target is 10 METs per week for basic fitness.

So, in rank order, some of the more obvious exercise regimes are as follows:

Activity	Intensity	METs per hour
Watching TV	As hard as you like	1
Walking	3 mph/ 5 kph	3
Walking Briskly	4 mph/ 6.4 kph	5
Resistance based gym work		6
Cycling	10-12 mph/ 16-19 kph	6
Team sports	Competitive	7
Boot Camp / Calisthenics	Vigorous	8
Swimming laps	Moderate	8
Tennis	Singles	8
Running	5 mph/ 8 kph	8
Cycling	14-16 mph/ 22-26 kph	9
Running	6 mph/ 10kph	10

Appendix 2

The business approach explained

It wasn't until after I'd written the first draft of the book that I realised that many of the concepts I had been using on a daily basis in my business life had helped my thinking in developing the "Life of Riley" habits.

For people totally uninterested in business this appendix won't be much worth reading, but some people are, I know, intensely interested in the subject. For them here is a bit of background on some of the business techniques I have borrowed for the book.

1 – Modelling

Building a good business model to justify an investment in a new product, or the purchase of a company, is a real skill. Making the model replicate what goes on in the real world needs a combination of great numeric/analytical skills, combined with a sophisticated understanding of what happens in markets when you make adjustments to the costs of production, the marketing or the pricing of the goods or services you offer.

Of course it's always possible to make a model turn a profit by making unrealistic assumptions (about cost-cutting, or sales uptake for example), so there's nothing more satisfactory than getting the model to "work" (i.e. produce a positive real return) without putting in assumptions that you know your more sceptical colleagues are going to rip to shreds.

When the model I developed for this book produced a highly significant correlation with the ONS data, I must admit I did feel the same sense of satisfaction I get when a business model tells me there's a good deal to be done.

2 – Research

Most businesses these days run on research and data. Whole departments are staffed with bright data managers crunching numbers to give their bosses an insight in to how people are thinking and acting. Products are launched only after the most extensive testing. Hugely expensive marketing campaigns can be ditched overnight if the attitudinal scores from test groups come back negative.

And these research groups aren't conducted randomly. As I mentioned earlier, the population is very carefully segmented before a single question is asked.

The marketeers know who you are, and they're coming after you, whether you like it or not.

3 – Continuous improvement

One theory which is a mainstay at business school is "kaizen".

This is the concept of "marginal gains". Making every step in the process just a tiny bit more efficient can lead to huge overall improvements.

This approach was pioneered by Japanese business after the end of WW2, and the rise of giant Japanese companies like Toyota, Sony et al was due to the relentless implementation of this theory – in part because of the influence of some pioneering American management consultants, including the revered W. Edwards Deming.

More recently it has been used in the world of sport – perhaps in the UK most famously by Sir Dave Brailsford in his work with the UKs cycling squads, and then Team Sky.

4 – Long term investment, compound

interest and tax planning

There's not much from a business perspective that is directly related to stopping smoking, but there are some financial implications it is worth pulling across from business to illustrate the benefits of stopping.

If you are a 20 a day smoker aged 34 (which is when I quit), stopping, and shifting that £8 per day cash into a pension instead could give you a huge financial return.

Thinking in terms of pensions isn't top of mind for most people in their 20s and 30s, but it should be, because long term financial planning benefits hugely from a concept known as compound interest. This is the idea that if you leave your cash invested in something that is adding interest (or growing in value if it's a stock for example) over a long period of time, the compounding effect of the interest growing on top of your original (and subsequent) investments can become hugely valuable.

The other business mainstay that carries across is looking for the best tax planning for any investment – and for you as an individual that will almost certainly be in your pension.

So, if you are spending £240 per month on cigarettes (£8 x 30 days) you could instead invest £300 from your pre-tax income in a pension and not be any worse off in your wallet or purse. If you did that every month for the 36 years until you were 70 (assuming you invested in stocks like a FTSE tracker fund growing at 7% per annum, and inflation was around 2%, both reasonable assumptions) that would create a pension pot of around a third of a million pounds – in today's money! That's a great ROI (Return On Investment – the holy grail for business plans!)

It might even be worth more because most companies will do some form of matching investment. Even if they just added a further 50% to your investment, that would nudge your pension pot to £500k in today's money. Half a million quid. That's a lot of reasons to give up the cigs.

5 – Return On Investment (ROI)

Of all the measures of business success there are, ROI is probably the most important. Businesspeople, financiers, entrepreneurs – all are searching for the best ROI, whether they are planning a new investment in their existing business, lending money to a start-up, or buying a company. Everything normally boils down to this. What return am I going to get for my money? If I put £1 into something, and only get 2p or 3p a year back, I might as well have left it in the bank. If I only get 6p or 7p, I might as well have put it in the stock market and forgotten about it.

Most professionals are looking for double digit returns – i.e. for every £1 they invest, they want an investment to pay at least a return of 12p-15p a year, or more. This is certainly the case within existing businesses, looking to invest their own cash in, say, a new product or a new factory.

Banks lending to established businesses might expect 5%-10% annual returns, but financiers lending to riskier businesses or newer start-ups might expect returns of 20%.

In fact, in the world of Private Equity, where whole firms are being purchased, the PE partners will normally expect a return of 30p or more every year for each pound they invest, although they might normally expect to get this return by selling the business for more than their purchase price at a later date, rather than taking money out each year.

And there's a good reason for looking for these higher returns. Two reasons in fact. The first is they are going to have to work at the investment, taking time and energy away from other activities (this is known as the Opportunity Cost). And secondly, and perhaps more importantly, putting money into businesses is risky. Overall, Private Equity only earns 15%-20% per annum across the industry over time because not every business they invest in makes it. So the stakes are high. By the way, these people are investing your money, if you have a pension, so we ought to be cheering them on if they deliver good returns for us (capitalist rant over).

Entrepreneurs, who are staking their own money, will want even higher returns for the same reasons.

And this is where you and I come in. For any plan for increasing life expectancy to be effective, its ROI must be spectacular, because a) it's our own time, effort and resource that we are going to expend, so there is an Opportunity Cost involved in taking us away from other activities (such as lazing on the couch, eating chocolate and drinking wine!), and b) it's risky because, through no fault of our own, we could get knocked over by the proverbial bus, effectively reducing our investment to nought! For many people, this fatalistic view of life is their default mode (what's the point of exercising, if I'm still likely to die in my 70s, is an often heard refrain).

Luckily, I think by now I've established that the returns, in terms of 10 to 15 years of extra life (with nearly all of it really healthy life too if the data is correct) are pretty spectacular, and the odds on being knocked over by that bus are pretty small. We just need now to ensure the investment isn't so large as to make even this sky-high return not worth the bother.

In order to do that, we need to ensure the plan itself is straightforward, and most importantly, easy, for us to implement. Only then will our ROI be truly spectacular.

6 – The Key Performance Indicator (KPI)

Every business will have these – a few measures of performance that the Board of Directors and senior managers will obsess over. And rightly so, if the numbers have been well chosen, and really do indicate the health of the company. Normally a KPI will be reported on daily, weekly or monthly, and the executive team will report the number itself, how it has moved since last reported, and whether it is closer or further away from a pre-specified goal which the Board have agreed. For a retailer, footfall might be a key measure, for a manufacturing company one KPI might be the amount of time a production line has been "down" for maintenance, or the amount of their cash stored up in "work in progress" on the factory floor. For a radio station like the ones I've run success might be defined by the size of your audience in the key demographic you are targeting, or the number of clients who return year on year to do business with you, or the number of spots you are able to sell every hour.

You can see why they vary from business to business, and why they become so important to monitor.

Appendix 3

Four week plan – for two people

Here's our plan for a typical month's eating – so there are four lots of four healthy meat/fish + vegetable recipes here for you to try. They are all really simple but very tasty and filling. I've suggested a standard salad to go with most of them – but feel free to experiment if you have other salad favourites you want to try – both in terms of veggie ingredients and flavourings. Just be careful not to stick in really unhealthy pre-prepared salad dressings.

Week 1
Monday: Cajun chicken with salad and quinoa
Tuesday: Salmon in coconut milk with salad and
             asparagus
Wednesday: Fillet steak with salad and grilled tomatoes
Thursday: Tuna steak with salad

Week 2
Monday: Turkey (or beef) mince chilli
Tuesday: Sea bass with wilted spinach and green beans
Wednesday: Chicken curry with lentil dhal
Thursday: Prawn stir-fry with cashew nuts

Week 3
Monday: Black bean chicken with bok choi and leeks
Tuesday: Baked salmon steaks with tomatoes
Wednesday: Sliced steak with rocket and salad
Thursday: Roasted cod with tomatoes

Week 4

Monday:	Roast chicken with veggies
Tuesday:	Swordfish with tomatoes, lemon and capers
Wednesday:	Chicken laksa
Thursday:	Pan fried trout with almonds & stir-fried vegetables

1 – Cajun Chicken with Salad and Quinoa

Ingredients:

400g pack of chicken breasts (2 to 3 breasts)
Cajun Spices (sold in most supermarket spice racks)
1 bag of lettuce
handful of cherry tomatoes, halved
1 red pepper, chopped into slices
1 green pepper, chopped into slices
1 avocado, peeled and cut into bite sized pieces
 (or feta cheese if you prefer)
50g quinoa
Extra virgin olive oil
Balsamic vinegar

Method:

Trim and slice the chicken breasts horizontally so they are thinner – they will grill more quickly. Gently score each side. Sprinkle a good helping of Cajun spices and olive oil over the chicken breasts and leave to marinade.

Heat a frying pan/griddle to a high heat (I use a griddle to add a nice scoring to the cooked meat) and grill the breasts for approximately 5-6 minutes each side, until they are fully cooked.

Add 50g of quinoa to 1 litre of boiling water, simmer for 10-12 minutes, then drain and run through a sieve to drain off any excess water.

Whilst the chicken is grilling, place the lettuce in a salad bowl. Add the halved cherry tomatoes, chopped and sliced peppers and either some avocado or feta cheese. Add some olive oil & balsamic vinegar (3 to 1 ratio) to flavour the salad. Finally, add the quinoa and mix the salad thoroughly.

2 – Salmon in Coconut Milk with Salad and Asparagus

Ingredients:

2 decently sized salmon fillets (150g-200g each)
2 chillies
400ml tin of coconut milk
200g asparagus
Extra virgin olive oil/toasted sesame oil

Method:

Place the 2 salmon fillets in an oven-proof dish. Cut the chillies in half length-wise, and scrape out the seeds using a teaspoon. Discard the seeds. Chop the chillies into smaller pieces and scatter over the salmon (being careful not to touch your eyes in the process). You can leave out the chillies if you are not a fan, but they do add a nice touch of extra flavour to the salmon.

Pour over the tin of coconut milk. Place in a pre-heated oven at 180°C with a lid on the dish (or some aluminium foil) and cook for 12-15 minutes – returning after 6 minutes to baste the fillets with the coconut milk.

Prepare a salad as per recipe 1.

Fry the asparagus for 2-3 minutes in either olive oil or sesame oil.

Serve the salmon with some of the remaining coconut milk drizzled over as a sauce.

3 – Fillet Steak with Grilled Tomatoes and Salad

Ingredients:

2 x 200-250g fillet steaks (8 oz each)
Salad ingredients as per recipe 1
2-3 large tomatoes
Extra virgin olive oil/butter

Method:

Bash the steaks with a rolling pin to flatten and tenderise them. Season the steaks with some milled pepper and a pinch of salt well rubbed in to both sides.

Pre-heat a frying pan/griddle. Again a griddle is better as it gets hotter and leaves that nice scoring effect on the surface of the steak. Add a touch of olive oil or butter to the griddle/pan and place the steaks on to cook. Allow 5 to 6 minutes per side depending on whether you want the steaks rare or medium and how thick they are. Take off the griddle/pan, place on a plate, and leave to continue cooking in their own juices for two to three minutes.

Cut the tomatoes in half, and place on the still hot pan/griddle cut side down to grill for 2 to 3 minutes.

Serve with a salad and some good English mustard.

Red Wine Sauce:

As an alternative to mustard you could make a red wine sauce. It will take longer than the steaks so start this first.

Chop an onion and fry it in some olive oil for 10 minutes, adding some garlic (I use the cheat's garlic you can buy, ready chopped) towards the end. Add a tin of chopped tomatoes, 250ml of red wine, and 500ml of chicken stock or bouillon. Bring to the boil and then simmer for 10 minutes.

Then strain the liquid to get rid of the onions and residual tomato pips etc, leaving you with just the strained liquid. Continue to simmer this until the liquid has reduced to a smooth sauce (maybe 15-20 minutes or so).

4 – Tuna Steak with Salad

Ingredients:

2 x 200g tuna Steaks
Salad ingredients
Mayonnaise
1 orange

Method:

Pre-heat your griddle or frying pan. Drizzle a little olive oil over when hot. Pan fry/griddle the tuna steaks for approximately 3 minutes on each side.

Prepare a salad as per recipe 1 (or make your own).

Take a small bowlful of mayonnaise, and whisk in the juice of an orange (or you could use lemon or lime if you prefer).

Serve the griddled/pan-fried tuna with the salad and the orange mayo side dressing for flavour. Add some side vegetables as well if you want.

5 – Turkey (or Beef) Mince Chilli

Ingredients:

400g turkey or beef mince
1 x 400gtin of chopped tomatoes
1 x 400g tin of kidney beans (with chilli sauce – check no added sugar)
1 x 400g tin of mixed beans
2 chillies, finely chopped (or 2 teaspoons pre-chopped chillies)
1 onion, finely chopped
2 cloves garlic (or 2 teaspoons pre-chopped garlic)
200ml red wine
1 cauliflower
Standard salad ingredients

Method:

Fry the chopped onion in olive oil until nicely soft and golden. Just at the end add the garlic and chillies and quickly fry with the browned onion.

Add the beef or turkey mince and fry until browned all over. Add the tomatoes, kidney beans and mixed beans, along with the red wine. Mix thoroughly and place in a lidded oven-proof dish and place in a pre-heated oven at 180°C for 30 minutes, until the chilli is fully cooked.

Take the white florets from a cauliflower, place in a food mixer and grind until the cauliflower has been reduced to rice-sized pellets (or a little smaller probably). Gently fry the cauliflower rice in butter for 6-8 minutes until soft and tender.

Serve the chilli with the cauliflower rice and a nice fresh green salad.

6 – Sea Bass with Wilted Spinach and Green Beans

Ingredients:

2 whole sea bass (filleted) or 4 fillets
300g bag of spinach
1 x 200g pack green beans
Juice of 1 lemon
25g butter
Olive oil
25g plain flour

Method:

Take the bag of spinach and sauté with some butter in a large frying pan or large saucepan. You will be amazed how quickly it shrinks – hence the big bag requirement. Once it has fully wilted place half on each plate.

Coat the sea bass / fillets with the flour, and fry in a hot pan in a little olive oil or butter for 2-3 minutes each side. If you are just doing the fillets fry the skin side first.

Separately blanch/boil the green beans (or you could use asparagus or sugar snap peas if you prefer) for 1-2 minutes until cooked but still with a bite to the taste.

Pour the juice of a lemon into a saucepan, heat until simmering and then add the butter in slices and mix thoroughly, adding more butter until you have a thick lemon butter sauce.

Place the fish over the wilted spinach, pour over the lemon butter and serve with your green vegetables.

7 – Chicken Curry with Lentil Dhal

Ingredients:

400g chicken breast (2-3 breasts), cut into small bite-sized pieces
2 onions, finely chopped
2 x 400g tins of chopped tomatoes
200ml can of coconut milk
100g red lentils

Spices:

1 tsp ground cumin
1 tsp ground coriander
1 tsp turmeric
2 sticks of lemongrass
400ml can of coconut cream
1 tbs fish sauce
2 tbs chillies (I keep a jar of easy, ready chopped chillies in the fridge)
2 tbs garlic (again, I keep a jar of easy, ready chopped garlic in the fridge)
2 tbs channa dhal spice (most Asian convenience stores will sell packs of this)
1 bunch of fresh coriander
2-3 star anise

Method:

Put the lentils into a saucepan and run through cold water until all the starch has been washed off and the water is clear. Cover the lentils with water and bring to the boil.

Fry 1 onion until soft, add a tin of chopped tomatoes, a teaspoonful each of chopped garlic and chopped chillies, and two teaspoons of the channa dhal mixture. Mix thoroughly and add to the boiling lentils. Keep simmering this mixture for an hour, adding a little water, until the lentils are soft to the bite.

Meanwhile, fry the other onion until soft. Add the chicken and fry until the pieces are beginning to turn brown. Add a teaspoon each of ground cumin, ground coriander and turmeric, along with the second tin of chopped tomatoes, and mix thoroughly.

In a food processor, place the lemongrass, a big handful of the fresh coriander, the fish sauce, another spoonful of garlic and chillies, a touch of olive oil and the coconut cream. Blend until it is a smooth paste.

Add the paste to the chicken and stir thoroughly. Add 2-3 star anise pods to the chicken and leave to simmer for 15-20 minutes.

Serve the chicken with the dhal. You could prepare some cauliflower rice to accompany the dish (see recipe 5).

8 – Prawn Stir-Fry with Cashew Nuts

Ingredients:

1 bag of pre-prepared vegetable stir-fry (most supermarkets sell these)
300g raw, shell-off prawns
50g cashew nuts
Sesame oil
1 tsp teaspoon of honey
3 tsp of soy sauce
2 tsp chopped garlic

Method:

Roast the cashew nuts in the sesame oil in a wok until golden, and then set aside.

Marinade the prawns in the honey, soy sauce and garlic for 30 minutes.

Toss the vegetable stir-fry inside the wok until the vegetables are hot and cooked (3-4 minutes). Quickly add the prawns and a dash more sesame oil to the wok and stir-fry until they turn pink and cooked (less than 1 minute). Add the cashews and serve. Again the cauliflower rice would go well with this.

9 – Black Bean Chicken with Bok Choi and Leeks

Ingredients:

400g chicken, cut into bite sized pieces
1 pack of bok choi (sometimes called pak choi or pak choy)
1 large leek
50g cashew nuts
½ x 200ml jar of black bean sauce
Sesame oil

Method:

Fry the cashew nuts in sesame oil for 2-3 minutes, until they start to look golden brown. Set to one side.

Stir fry the chicken pieces in sesame oil until browned all over. Set to one side.

Chop the bok choi/pak choi into small slices, discarding the hard end. Similarly slice the leek in half length-wise, and slice into 1/4-inch segments. Stir-fry the leeks and bok choi in sesame oil until softened. Add the chicken, cashew nuts and the black bean sauce, and stir-fry until everything is nicely mixed and covered in the sauce.

Serve on its own, or with the cauliflower rice referred to earlier.

Note: this is one recipe where I have suggested you buy a shop-prepared sauce – black bean sauce is possible to make yourself but is a bit of a faff compared to buying a jar of sauce, and the amount of sauce needed won't spoil any nutritional goals.

10 – Baked Salmon Steaks with Tomatoes

Ingredients:

2 large salmon steaks (200g each)
1 pack of vine tomatoes
1 pepper, thinly sliced
1 leek, halved and chopped
1 lemon, sliced
1 pack of asparagus (100g) (or green beans, mange tout etc.)
Olive oil
200ml white wine
2 tsp of chopped chillies

Method:

Place the salmon steaks in an oven-proof dish. Drizzle with olive oil and the chopped chillies. Slice the lemon and place the slices on top of the salmon. Place the vine tomatoes on top and surrounding the steaks, along with the pepper, cut into slices, and the chopped leeks. Add sufficient white wine to give the dish enough juice to cook in – especially the vegetables.

Place in a pre-heated oven at 180°C in a lidded dish and cook for 25-30 minutes.

Stir-fry the asparagus (or other small green vegetables) in some olive oil for 2-3 minutes, until still crunchy but nicely cooked.

Serve the salmon steaks with the cooked veg and asparagus.

11 – Sliced Steak with Rocket and Salad

Ingredients:

400g of fillet steak
1 big bag of rocket
Peppers
Tomatoes
Avocado
50g quinoa, boiled and strained
½ cucumber
1 tbs lemon juice
1 tsp honey
1 tsp English mustard
Olive oil

Method:

Prepare the steak as if you were cooking it in the previous steak recipe, and griddle/stir-fry as before – 5 minutes+ each side. Once fully cooked, slice the steaks thinly and place on a bed of rocket on each plate.

Separately, prepare a salad of chopped peppers, chopped tomatoes, a thinly chopped avocado, a peeled, seeded and chopped cucumber, mixed with 50g of quinoa that has been boiled/strained.

Make a vinaigrette using a tablespoon of lemon, tablespoon of olive oil, a teaspoon of English mustard and a teaspoon of honey. This adds a lovely flavour to the salad.

Serve on the side of the steak/rocket with a dab of English mustard.

12 – Roasted Cod with Tomatoes

Ingredients:

2 skinless cod fillets (about 200g per person)
1 red pepper, chopped
1 red onion, chopped
125g cherry tomatoes
1 jar of smooth tomato paste (passata)
1 small bunch of basil
Standard salad ingredients

Method:

Pre-heat the oven to 200°C. Place the chopped peppers, tomatoes and onion in an oven-proof dish, sprinkle some olive oil and pepper on top and cook for 15 minutes until beginning to char.

Place the cod fillets in the dish alongside the charred veg, pour over the passata and place in the oven for a further 15 minutes until cooked. Sprinkle the basil on top.

Serve with a green salad.

13 – Roast Chicken with Veggies

Ingredients:

1 small chicken for roasting (1Kg to 1.5Kg)
1 lemon, ended and halved
1 red pepper
1 green pepper
1 red onion
Handful of cherry tomatoes, halved
150g cauliflower
150g broccoli
25g butter,
25g plain flour
500 ml milk
75g grated cheddar cheese

Method:

Place half the lemon inside the chicken. Score the outside of the chicken lightly, and rub over with the juice of the other half of the lemon and some olive oil (and possibly some chopped chillies/garlic if you like those flavours). Place in a roasting tray and roast for 20 minutes in a pre-heated oven at 220°C and then a further 40 minutes per kg on a reduced temperature of 180°C.

Separately place the chopped peppers, onion and cherry tomatoes in a small oven-proof dish, drizzle with olive oil and season with some pepper.

Make the cheese sauce. Melt the butter in a saucepan, stir in the flour. Cook for 1-2 minutes. Stir in the milk until you have a smooth sauce. Simmer for around 5 to 6 minutes. Add the grated cheese until thoroughly mixed into the sauce and melted but let it cool as it does so.

Break the cauliflower and broccoli into small florets, and pour over the cheese sauce.

When there is about 10 minutes to go in the oven for the chicken, place the veggies in.

Take the chicken out and then place the cauliflower/broccoli cheese in and cook for 20 minutes.

Let the chicken cool down, carve, and serve with the roasted veggies and cauliflower/broccoli cheese.

You may end up with more chicken than you need for one meal for two people - so save the remainder in the fridge to add to a salad.

14 – Swordfish with Tomatoes, Lemon & Capers

Ingredients:

2 x 200g swordfish steaks
2 bunches of vine tomatoes
1 lemon
Olive oil
Mint and basil leaves
Handful of capers
Salad ingredients

Method:

Make an olive oil/lemon mix (3 tablespoons each), and add in some chopped basil and mint leaves (a handful of each). Then add a little pepper to season. Baste each side of the swordfish steaks with the olive oil/lemon sauce.

Pre-heat your griddle or frying pan. Drizzle a little olive oil over when hot. Pan fry/griddle the swordfish steaks for approximately 3 minutes on each side.

Pop the vine tomatoes in the pan to warm and cook alongside the swordfish. Pop the capers in towards the end to warm through too.

Serve the swordfish with the vine tomatoes on top and the capers added on the side for flavour/bite.

Prepare a salad as per recipe 1 (or make your own) to go with the fish.

15 – Chicken Laksa

Ingredients:

2-3 chicken breasts, sliced lengthways
1 x 400ml can of coconut milk
fresh green beans (or okra) and halved cherry tomatoes for
the side
1 chopped chilli
Cauliflower rice (see recipe 5)

For the sauce:

2 sticks of lemongrass, ended and peeled
2 tsp of chopped chillies
2 tsp turmeric
handful of fresh coriander
handful of fresh mint
½ tsp shrimp paste
1 tsp fish sauce
2 tbs of sesame oil

Method:

Place the strips of chicken on a griddle (or in a frying pan)
and fry/griddle, turning constantly, until they are nicely
cooked and browned. Remove and on a chopping board, cut
into small, bite-sized pieces.

Separately, mix the sauce ingredients in a blender, and blend
until you have formed a smooth paste.

Fry the paste quickly in a frying pan, then add the coconut
milk and the chicken pieces and thoroughly warm through.

Separately fry the green beans (or chopped okra – cut into ½
inch segments) in some sesame oil with a teaspoon of
chillies and the cherry tomatoes for a couple of minutes until
cooked but still crunchy (the okra will be softer if you do
that instead).

Serve the laksa over some cauliflower rice with the green beans/okra on the side.

16 – Pan-fried trout with almonds & stir-fried vegetables

Ingredients:

4 trout fillets
1 lemon, quartered
1 bag of flaked almonds
1 bag of stir-fry vegetables
25g plain flour
Olive oil

Method:

Dry toast the flaked almonds in a frying pan until golden brown. Set aside.

Lightly dust the trout fillets with some flour. Fry in olive oil for 2-3 minutes each side until cooked.

Separately, stir fry the vegetables in some sesame oil.

Serve the trout with the almonds sprinkled on top, and some lemon juice squeezed over for some bite, with the stir-fry on the side.

References

Note: Correct as of original publication date.

[i] http://io9.com/i-fooled-millions-into-thinking-chocolate-helps-weight-1707251800

[ii] http://www.ons.gov.uk/ons/rel/vsob1/mortality-statistics--deaths-registered-in-england-and-wales--series-dr-/2010/stb-deaths-by-cause-2010.html

[iii] http://www.bris.ac.uk/social-community-medicine/projects/caerphilly/

[iv] http://www.alcohollearningcentre.org.uk/Topics/Browse/BriefAdvice/?parent=4444&child=4896

[v] http://www.britishlivertrust.org.uk/

[vi] http://www.britishlivertrust.org.uk/liver-information/liver-conditions/non-alcoholic-fatty-liver-disease/

[vii] https://www.drinkaware.co.uk/make-a-change/how-to-cut-down/take-a-break-from-alcohol/

[viii] http://www.ons.gov.uk/ons/rel/ghs/opinions-and-lifestyle-survey/adult-smoking-habits-in-great-britain--2013/stb-opn-smoking-2013.html

[ix] http://www.theguardian.com/society/2014/feb/26/social-smokers-underestimate-risks-study

[x] http://jama.jamanetwork.com/article.aspx?articleid=1555137

[xi] http://www.noo.org.uk/uploads/doc/vid_7199_Obesity_and_life_expectancy.pdf

[xii] http://www.thetimes.co.uk/tto/health/news/article4267077.ece?shareToken=a2e50a18a64fb52d02e2c5291ee77f5a

xiii http://www.hscic.gov.uk/catalogue/PUB13218/HSE2012-Ch10-Adult-BMI.pdf

xiv http://easo.org/perception-survey/summary-of-all-countries/survey-uk/

xvhttp://www.kcl.ac.uk/newsevents/news/newsrecords/2015/July/Lowchanceofrecoveringnormalbodyweight.aspx

xvi
http://www.cmaj.ca/content/early/2015/11/23/cmaj.150535.full.pdf

xvii http://www.hscic.gov.uk/catalogue/PUB13648/Obes-phys-acti-diet-eng-2014-rep.pdf

xviii http://www.ijbnpa.org/content/5/1/56

xix http://www.bristol.ac.uk/media-library/sites/cmpo/migrated/documents/wp311.pdf

xx http://www.ncbi.nlm.nih.gov/pmc/articles/PMC3501820/

xxi http://www.thelancet.com/journals/lancet/article/PIIS0140-6736%2811%2960749-6/abstract

xxii http://www.ons.gov.uk/ons/rel/mortality-ageing/mortality-in-england-and-wales/average-life-span/rpt-average-life-span.html#tab-Trends-in-Average-Life-Span

xxiii http://understandinguncertainty.org/why-life-expectancy-misleading-summary-survival

xxiv http://www.kingsfund.org.uk/time-to-think-differently/trends/demography/life-expectancy#healthy

xxv http://www.thetimes.co.uk/tto/health/news/article4443070.ece

xxvi http://www.hscic.gov.uk/catalogue/PUB10932

xxvii http://www.hscic.gov.uk/catalogue/PUB10932

xxviii http://velvetgloveironfist.blogspot.co.uk/2015/07/the-middle-class-drink-epidemic.html

xxixhttp://www.theguardian.com/society/2015/may/22/alcohol-consumption-in-england-is-underestimated-says-study xxx http://www.thetimes.co.uk/tto/health/dr-mark-porter/article4270324.ece?shareToken=a5b0894a393173f2236cb74ce423d5f5

xxxi http://www.ncbi.nlm.nih.gov/pubmed/23072405

xxxii http://www.cdc.gov/tobacco/data_statistics/fact_sheets/health_effects/tobacco_related_mortality/

xxxiii http://www.anu.edu.au/news/all-news/almost-two-million-smokers-will-die-from-their-habit

xxxiv http://www.ncbi.nlm.nih.gov/pmc/articles/PMC1488756/

xxxv http://archive.sportengland.org/research/active_people_survey/active_people_survey_7.aspx

xxxvi http://news.harvard.edu/gazette/story/2012/11/how-much-exercise-is-enough/

xxxvii http://www.hindawi.com/journals/jar/2012/243958/

xxxviii http://understandinguncertainty.org/what-your-effective-age

xxxix http://www.kcl.ac.uk/ioppn/news/records/2015/August/ecigarettes.aspx

xl http://www.nytimes.com/2015/04/17/health/use-of-e-cigarettes-rises-sharply-among-teenagers-report-says.html?smid=tw-share&_r=0

xli http://www.nejm.org/doi/full/10.1056/NEJMoa1414293#t=article

xlii http://www.thelancet.com/journals/lancet/article/PIIS0140-6736%2812%2961720-6/abstract

xliii http://www.ncbi.nlm.nih.gov/pmc/articles/PMC1447499/

xliv http://www.dailymail.co.uk/health/article-1350351/Trying-quit-smoking-It-years-seven-attempts.html

xlv http://www.hsph.harvard.edu/news/press-releases/more-whole-grains-linked-with-lower-mortality-risk/

xlvi

http://www.maastrichtuniversity.nl/web/Main/Sitewide/News1/Daily
ConsumptionOfNutsAndPeanutsLinkedToLowerMortalityRates1.htm

xlvii http://www.theguardian.com/society/2015/aug/30/brisk-daily-
walks-reduce-ageing-increase-life-span-research

xlviii http://www.ncbi.nlm.nih.gov/pubmed/10422091

xlix http://newsroom.heart.org/news/moderate-coffee-drinking-may-be-
linked-to-reduced-risk-of-death?preview=7525

l https://blogs.ucl.ac.uk/hbrc/2012/06/29/busting-the-21-days-habit-
formation-myth/

li

http://www.thetimes.co.uk/tto/opinion/columnists/article4449967.ece

lii

http://www.thetimes.co.uk/tto/health/news/article4435056.ece?share
Token=1d56f46343149ef8ab6d9707e2fb623a

liii http://mobile.nytimes.com/2015/04/21/upshot/simple-habits-for-
healthy-eating.html?referrer

liv http://www.acc.org/about-acc/press-
releases/2015/01/13/11/50/for-most-healthy-obese-health-declines-
over-time

lv http://jama.jamanetwork.com/article.aspx?articleid=1730520

lvi http://www.theguardian.com/lifeandstyle/2015/oct/30/low-fat-
diets-slammed-major-new-report?CMP=edit_2221

lvii http://www.zoeharcombe.com/

lviii

http://corporate.dukemedicine.org/news_and_publications/news_office
/news/7598

lix http://authoritynutrition.com/23-studies-on-low-carb-and-low-fat-
diets/

lx http://www.cell.com/cell-metabolism/abstract/S1550-
4131(12)00189-1

lxi http://www.nytimes.com/2015/08/30/opinion/diet-advice-that-ignores-hunger.html?smprod=nytcore-ipad&smid=nytcore-ipad-share

lxii http://www.theguardian.com/society/2015/mar/16/the-next-aa-moderation-management-abstinence-alcohol-isnt-the-answer?CMP=share_btn_link

lxiii http://www.bmj.com/content/309/6959/911

lxiv http://velvetgloveironfist.blogspot.co.uk/2015/04/tim-stockwell-merchant-of-doubt.html

lxv http://understandinguncertainty.org/misleading-conclusions-alcohol-protection-study

lxvi http://archinte.jamanetwork.com/article.aspx?articleid=769554

lxvii http://onlinelibrary.wiley.com/doi/10.1111/j.1530-0277.2010.01286.x/abstract

lxviii
http://archinte.jamanetwork.com/article.aspx?articleid=769554#tab

lxix http://www.ncbi.nlm.nih.gov/pubmed/20626370

lxx http://velvetgloveironfist.blogspot.co.uk/2016/01/a-crucial-point-about-alcohol-research.html

lxxi http://now.tufts.edu/news-releases/walking-faster-or-longer-linked-significant-cardiovascular-benefits-older-adults

lxxii http://news.harvard.edu/gazette/story/2012/11/how-much-exercise-is-enough/

lxxiii http://bjsm.bmj.com/content/49/11/743

lxxiv http://jech.bmj.com/content/57/6/440.full

lxxv
http://www.noo.org.uk/uploads/doc/vid_16966_AdultSocioeconSep2012.pdf

lxxvi http://www.hscic.gov.uk/article/6878/One-in-four-affluent-adults-drink-above-lower-risk-levels lxxvii

https://www.york.ac.uk/media/economics/documents/herc/wp/05_02.pdf

lxxviii http://www.thetimes.co.uk/tto/health/news/article4443070.ece

lxxix

http://www.kcl.ac.uk/newsevents/news/newsrecords/2015/January/Exercise-allows-you-to-age-optimally.aspx

lxxx http://www.ncbi.nlm.nih.gov/pubmed/18268169

lxxxi https://today.duke.edu/2015/04/arginine

lxxxii http://www.theguardian.com/society/2015/mar/12/dancing-sudoku-fish-and-fruit-the-keys-to-a-mentally-alert-old-age

lxxxiii http://www.nhs.uk/news/2015/03March/Pages/Diet-exercise-and-brain-training-may-help-keep-the-mind-sharp.aspx

lxxxiv

https://www.alzheimers.org.uk/site/scripts/news_article.php?newsID=2494

lxxxv http://jama.jamanetwork.com/article.aspx?articleid=199487

lxxxvi http://www.thelancet.com/journals/landia/article/PIIS2213-8587(15)00033-9/abstract

lxxxvii http://www.diabetes.co.uk/type3-diabetes.html

lxxxviii http://www.ons.gov.uk/ons/rel/lifetables/historic-and-projected-data-from-the-period-and-cohort-life-tables/2012-based/index.html

lxxxix http://techcrunch.com/2015/11/23/chaotic-moon-explores-biometric-tattoos-for-medicine-and-the-military/

xc

http://www.thetimes.co.uk/tto/news/uk/article4414041.ece?shareToken=a804d5b8410a92bdf6898c66c3a51ea8

xci http://www.ncbi.nlm.nih.gov/pubmed/26000489

xcii http://www.healthline.com/health-news/is-da-vinci-robotic-surgery-revolution-or-ripoff-021215#4 xciii http://www.theguardian.com/society/2015/jun/01/paradigm-shift-hailed-in-treatment-of-lung-cancer?CMP=twt_gu

xciv
http://www.sciencedaily.com/releases/2007/05/070503205701.htm

xcv http://www.theguardian.com/nanotechnology-world/nanotechnology-shaping-stem-cell-research

xcvi
http://www.rsc.org/chemistryworld/Issues/2010/July/BiomaterialsRevolution.asp

xcvii http://www.theguardian.com/science/shortcuts/2015/mar/18/of-mice-and-old-men-is-the-elixir-of-youth-finally-coming-of-age

xcviii http://visual.ons.gov.uk/what-are-your-chances-of-living-to-100/

Index

About the Author

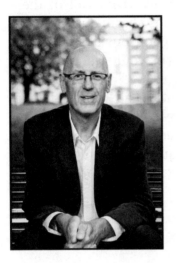

Phil Riley is an award-winning broadcaster and business executive.

In his early career he won the Japan Prize for educational broadcasting, before going on to earn an MBA from one of the world's leading business schools, at Columbia University in New York City, where he was placed in the Dean's Honor List every semester, and graduated Beta Gamma Sigma (the US equivalent of a 1st class honours degree).

In his subsequent career he has launched or relaunched some of the UK's most famous radio station brands (Heart, Magic and LBC are included on the list) and has made millions of pounds in profits for shareholders in his businesses throughout his career.

In 2013 he was named as one of the 40 most influential people in commercial radio's first 40 years, and in 2014 was given the prestigious Arqiva Special Award for his "life-long and continuing commitment to the medium of radio."

He has also been at various stages of his life a smoker, clinically obese, chronically unfit and a heavy/frequent drinker, and suffered a near-death experience in 2013.

Over time he has managed to overcome all of these challenges, and now, in this book, he is sharing his thoughts on how, by applying the basics of good business planning and management, you can transform your life by making some straightforward lifestyle changes.

The "Life of Riley" habits capture all of the changes required in one simple, easy to follow routine.

More than a diet, more than just an exercise schedule, the "Life of Riley" habits are a unique, total solution to the lifestyle challenges we all face, that can end up adding years to your life.